MOVEMENT
is
MEDICINE

The therapeutic effect of physical activity on mental health disorders in children and young people

Dr Sanjiv Nichani OBE

www.ukbookpublishing.com
ISBN: 978-1-918077-32-2

Contents

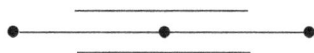

DR SANJIV NICHANI

OBE awarded for services to Medicine and Charity

Dr Sanjiv Nichani Senior Consultant Paediatrician Leicester Children's Hospital and Founder of Healing Little Hearts Global Foundation

Dr Nichani is a prolific national campaigner against what he calls the Screendemic has been featured as an expert in the Channel 4 documentary Swiped as well as BBC Morning Live. ITV Central News and a number of BBC radio stations such as BBCRadio4, BBC Five Live etc and has written nationally accepted guidelines on what is appropriate screen time for ages 0-17 years

Dr Nichani is also a long standing practitioner of Shotokan Karate and is a 5th Degree Black belt and practices the concept of Movement is Medicine himself.

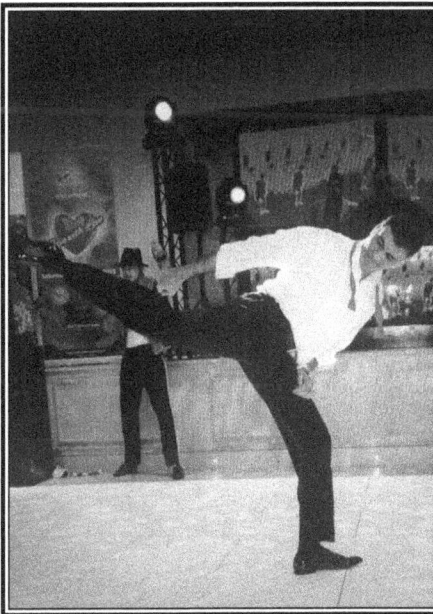

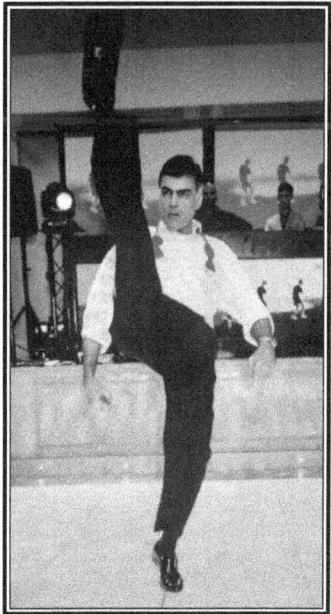

Dr Sanjiv Nichani OBE

CHAPTER 1

———•———•———•———

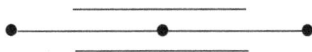

Setting the Scene/
The Background

In the last 15 years societies across the world are changing and evolving at a rapid pace.

This is nothing new for humanity; however, two things are different this time:

Firstly, the welcome and increased focus on mental health illness, reflective of a more holistic approach to an individual; and secondly, the massive change brought about by the Internet Revolution, more specifically the 24/7 Smartphone, Device and Social Media Use and of course more recently the dramatic arrival of AI.

As a result of the invasion of our lives by Smartphones, Devices and Social Media Apps in the last 15 years, civilisation as we know it has been upended completely.

Simultaneously, and perhaps emanating from the significant focus on mental health difficulties particularly in children, adolescents and young adults, there has been a huge increase in the diagnosis of Anxiety and Depression, ADHD and Autism etc amongst children and teenagers.

Now there is a currently an animated debate raging across the world as to whether there is a clear causal link between excessive screen time, social media use and the collapse of mental health well-being amongst children and adolescents.

There are opposing sides of academics squaring up against each other deliberating whether the advent of the 24/7 ubiquitous Internet use has a causal role in the epidemic of mental illness in the young.

I am sure you will agree with me that whatever side of the debate one is on, there must be unanimous agreement that spending hours and hours in front of smartphones or devices and social media apps at any age cannot be healthy for the individual, and given the number of people around the world who are addicted to smartphones, devices and social media apps, for the human race as a whole.

The 24/7 connectivity has entrapped huge swathes of the world's population and irrevocably changed the behaviour of millions of people.

A revolution that started out in order to facilitate interaction and connection between human beings, which purported to allow that regardless of the distance between people, has instead lured large sections of the population into addictive behaviours, imprisoned by and enslaved to a virtual world that bears no resemblance to and actually completely distorts the real world and its realities.

As humanity is learning at great cost with global warming, going against the grain of nature comes at a huge price.

In the case of global warming, that price is calamitous destruction of the ecosystems of the planet whilst in the virtual world it is the tragic destruction of human interaction as we know it.

In this case we have gone against the laws of nature by substituting real life in-person communication with virtual societies with many aspects of these, so called virtual societies are becoming malevolent and antisocial.

As a result, we are now in the middle of a SCREEN DEMIC that has changed human beings beyond recognition.

The SCREEN DEMIC is the Epidemic of Mental Health Illness in Children, Teenagers and Young Adults, as well as difficulties in early language development and communication due to excessive screen time and social media use.

Adults are not immune to the SCREEN DEMIC, but children, due to their developing brains, are particularly vulnerable. With regards to adults, it is likely that the term digital dementia will make a regular appearance in the medical press in future.

In other words, adults who spend their entire working lives on screens, by necessity, as well as almost all of their recreational times on screens by choice, and do very little else, are at risk of brain changes as well as early onset dementia.

Now in my opinion the most accurate way to describe an issue or a problem is with the help of statistics so here are a few:

In the USA, people spend an average of five hours and 16 minutes per day on their phones, with Gen Z spending the most time on their phone, on average about six hours and 27 minutes, and Baby Boomers spending a little over four hours (which is still double the recommended limit).

In another recent US survey, children spent an average of 90 minutes out of a 6.5-hour school day on their phones. Regardless of your attitude towards technology, I hope you will agree that this represents an extraordinary waste of time and human potential.

Further statistics reveal that most Americans can't seem to put their phones down and are reaching for their device an average of 352 times a day, once every two minutes and 43 seconds –according to tech care company Asurion*. Whether we're sending text messages, capturing content or looking at reels, it's a nearly four-fold increase from a similar survey conducted by Asurion before the pandemic, in 2019, when Americans said they checked their phones 96 times a day**.

What about in the UK and indeed in the rest of the world?

The situation isn't much different; just look at the number of adults walking around with their phones buried in their heads: The Phombies.

Back to the stats: Teenagers in the UK are spending, on average, six hours and 39 minutes per day on screens. This includes time spent on social media, gaming, and texting, but **does not** include screen time for schoolwork or homework.

Make no mistake about it, these shocking statistics are evidence of an addiction to smartphones, devices and social media apps in 30-35% of teenagers in the UK.

The statistics for the rest of the English-speaking world are very similar and this dramatic increase in mental health difficulties amongst children and young people has been mirrored in Canada, Australia and New Zealand.

What about other parts of the globe?

Let's look at a study that will give us an idea:

Every three years, the Organisation for Economic Co-operation and Development (OECD) conducts an educational assessment (PISA) of students across 80 countries around the world.

Whilst 80 nation states does not include the entire world of nearly 200 countries, it is, nevertheless, a significant sample!

The PISA assessment focusses on Maths and Science, and the last assessment was published in December 2023.

I am going to focus on three key findings from this PISA assessment.

1. Since 2012, with the advent of Smartphones, Devices and Social Media Apps, grades have dropped progressively across all 80 countries!
2. Smartphones in class distract not only the child with the smartphone but also children around the person with the smartphone due to the fear of missing out.
3. When children do not have their smartphones on them they feel ill at ease, ie they feel a part of them or their being is missing.

In other words, children are growing up in a phone-based and a phone-controlled childhood, unlike the play-based childhood that previous generations of people grew up in.

More on the same theme.

Performance in reasoning and problem-solving tests has been declining among teenagers and adults since the early 2010s, when smartphones became widespread. Average IQ, which rose steadily throughout the 20th century, began to fall at about the same time. Reliance on AI, according to a recent Microsoft study, may be "slowly impairing our critical thinking skills".

A sober analysis of the data in the Financial Times concludes that we are witnessing an "erosion in the human ability for mental capacity and application".

Furthermore, an internal report produced by TikTok stated that regular use of the app leads to "loss of analytical skills, memory formation, contextual thinking, and conversational depth".

What about other aspects of smartphones and social media use?

Pressure on young people to live up to glamorous images of their friends on social media is leaving them feeling inadequate. There is an expectation that you should be beautiful and constantly enjoying yourself. That isn't real life, although it is portrayed as such, leading to people feeling inadequate and disappointed with low self-esteem.

I have listed a few more very well recognised and documented adverse effects below:

Social media can amplify the fear of missing out on social events and experiences, leading to anxiety (FOMO).

Anxiety and Depression Studies show a correlation between excessive social media use and increased rates of depression and anxiety among young people.

Cyberbullying:
Children and teens are vulnerable to cyberbullying on social media, which can cause significant psychological distress.

Decreased Social Skills:
Reduced face-to-face interactions due to increased reliance on virtual communication can hinder the development of social skills.

Academic Distraction:
Smartphones and social media can be a major distraction from schoolwork and studying, impacting academic performance as already highlighted.

Impaired Attention Span:
Frequent smartphone use can contribute to reduced attention spans and difficulties with focus and concentration.

Exposure to Unsuitable Content:
Children and teens are often exposed to inappropriate content online, including violence, pornography, and misinformation.

Risk of Online Predators:
Social media can expose young people to online predators who may try to exploit or extort them.

False Sense of Security:
Social media can create a false sense of security and lead to the sharing of too much personal information.

Sleep Disruption:
Using smartphones before bed can disrupt sleep patterns, impacting mood and cognitive function.

Reduced Physical Activity:
Excessive screen time can lead to a more sedentary lifestyle, potentially contributing to physical health problems.

Now if I have given you the impression that I am a luddite and anti-technology, then let me state emphatically that technology is now an integral part of our lives; however, lines have become blurred, meaning technology, ie smartphones and apps have gone from being used for functional purposes to being addictive.

I am vociferously against the current reality which is that for far too many children, adolescents, young and older adults, technology is in control rather than the other way round.

Children, young people and adults are living lives controlled by smartphones and social media apps at great cost and this Internet revolution is leading to Human Brain Involution.

The world is now finally waking up to the fact that the Screen Demic has engulfed humanity and there is a worldwide movement agitating about the adverse effects of Smartphone use in children and teenagers, and the damaging effects of social media on developing brains.

We all need to get smart about what these so-called smartphones are doing to our children and that the sequelae from social media is leading to countless antisocial effects.

The time to act is now as it is never too late and a ready-made and relatively simple action plan involves physical activity, which is the essence of this book.

Now, whilst I have spent a lot of this chapter talking about the Screen Demic, I have also devoted chapters in the book specifically focussing on other common mental health disorders in childhood, such as Anxiety and Depression, ADHD, Autistic Spectrum disorder, and Internet Gaming Disorder.

The increased awareness of all of these conditions is most welcome; however, due to the massive increase in diagnoses, the mental health services are being completely overwhelmed and overrun.

It is in that context that I am suggesting that you think of easy-to-do, accessible any time of the day or evening (within reason of course), economical and effective ways of managing children and adolescents with Mental Health Disorders: Physical Activity.

Through the next few chapters I am going to provide you with the scientific understanding of the structural and chemical abnormalities in the brains of children and teenagers with a variety of common mental health disorders, and also digestible evidence as to how physical activity helps and indeed reverses many of these abnormal brain changes.

That is the essence of Movement is Medicine: The Science behind the therapeutic effects of Physical Activity on children and adolescents with Mental Health Disorders.

CHAPTER 2

●————————●————————●

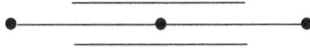

Brain Dynamics and Brain Neuroplasticity

The basic premise of my book, that physical activity can be therapeutic for children and teenagers with mental health disorders, is based on the existence of neuroplasticity.

Scientists have known about neuroplasticity for a long time, but fine details have emerged relatively recently, facilitated by incredible advances in medical technology and the ability to map brain activity.

Brain neuroplasticity in children and adolescents refers to the brain's remarkable ability to change, reorganise, and grow nerve cells and pathways in response to experiences, learning, and even injury.

Let me explain:

The brain has 100 billion neurons or nerve cells that are required for the brain to function in the way that we know it and in a manner that clearly separates us from the rest of the animal kingdom.

In fact, childhood in humans comprises the longest period of development in the entire animal kingdom, which highlights the hugely complex processes that are involved in brain maturation.

The fact that this process goes on for such a long period of time works to the advantage of individuals who have had health or social difficulties during a particular period in their developing years, ie there is scope to retrain and/or reorientate the brain due to this incredible feature of neuroplasticity.

The human brain undergoes rapid development in the early years of life. At birth, the brain is approximately 25% of its adult weight but achieves nearly 90% by age six (Lenroot & Giedd, 2006).

The Brain Builds in Layers

Think of your child's brain like a house under construction:
- The foundation (basic senses, movement) is laid early.
- The rooms and wiring (thinking, emotions) are added gradually.
- The control systems (judgment, planning, self-control) are finished last – in the teenage years and beyond.

At birth, a child's brain is a work in progress. It develops as they experience the world through seeing, hearing, tasting, touching, and smelling the environment.

The natural, simple, loving encounters between adults and children that occur throughout the day, such as a caregiver singing, smiling, talking to, and rocking their baby, are essential to this process. All of these encounters with the outside world affect the child's emotional development and shape how their brain becomes wired and how it will work.

- Positive experiences of babies as described above have long-lasting effects on their ability to learn and regulate their emotions. When there is an absence of appropriate teaching and interaction in the baby's environment, the brain's development can be affected and there are more likely to be sustained negative effects.
- When normal and active parental interaction with their children is substituted by significant amounts of time spent passively in front of a smartphone or a device, this can have severe detrimental effects on the child's development.

- On the other hand, if families provide ample learning opportunities and stimulation, they can facilitate brain development.
- Learning is about connection between the major nerve cells in the brain, the neurons. Neurons transmit information between each other through chemical and electrical signals via synapses or junctions thereby forming neural networks, a series of interconnected nerve cells.
- This is what is meant by "the wiring of the brain" and "neurons that fire together are wired together".

Nerve cells and junctions between nerve cells grow exponentially in the first years of life, even before a baby can walk and talk.

As an infant experiences something or learns something for the first time, a strong neural connection is made. If this experience is repeated, the connection is reactivated and becomes strengthened and gets embedded over time.

If the experience is not repeated, connections are reduced and removed.

In this way, the brain discards or "prunes" what is not necessary and consolidates the connections that are used frequently. During infancy and the first years of childhood, there is significant loss of nerve cell pathways as the brain starts to prune away or discard what it doesn't believe it will need to function.

This process of pruning is what makes the early years so important.

For instance, if a child's language centre is not stimulated by vocabulary from parents, siblings, friends and family, the pathways do not develop. This can then lead to the advent of non-verbal children.

Therefore, the earlier in a child's development that we provide varied learning experiences, the stronger those behaviours and skills are secured in the brain.

The brain's neuroplasticity not only allows it to reorganise pathways and create new connections, it also allows the brain to create new neurons.

There are two main types of neuroplasticity:
- Functional plasticity is the brain's ability to move functions from a damaged area of the brain to other undamaged areas.
- Structural plasticity is the brain's ability to actually change its physical structure as a result of learning.

Neurons that are used frequently develop stronger connections. Those that are rarely or never used eventually die. By developing new connections and pruning away weak ones, the brain can adapt to the changing environment. Crucially, these pathways can be reopened if consistent use or stimulation occurs subsequently.

Evidence: Experiences shape brain architecture by strengthening active synaptic connections, a phenomenon often described as "use it or lose it" (Shonkoff & Phillips, 2000).

Mechanisms of Neuroplasticity

Neuroplasticity in children is underpinned by a number of mechanisms:

Synaptic Plasticity

What Are Synapses?
Imagine your brain is like a huge city filled with roads. These roads are pathways between nerve cells (neurons). At the junctions where two neurons connect, there are synapses or tiny gaps where messages are passed from one neuron to another.

What Happens at a Synapse?

When a message travels through your brain – like when you're learning something new or remembering a fact – a small burst of chemicals (called neurochemicals) is released at the synapse. This helps the signal jump from one neuron to the next.

I'm delving into a bit more detail to further cement your understanding of neuroplasticity:

Long-Term Potentiation (LTP) – "Strengthening the Connection"
LTP is like upgrading a dirt road into a highway.

If two neurons frequently "talk" to each other (meaning they keep sending signals back and forth), due to repeated stimulation by a particular activity, the brain responds by making connections between the two neurons stronger and by an ongoing series of chemical processes, memories become embedded.

This is how you get better at things over time, like learning a language, playing piano, or remembering faces. LTP is thought to be the biological basis for learning and memory.

Long-Term Depression (LTD) – "Weakening the Connection"
LTD is like downgrading or closing a road that's rarely used.

If a connection between two neurons is used less often, the brain says "This connection isn't very useful. Let's scale it back."

So the synapse becomes weaker:

This helps the brain clear out unneeded or outdated information, making room for new learning. LTD is important for forgetting things you no longer need and for refining skills (like correcting a bad habit or relearning a task the right way – and goodness knows we all pick up bad habits along the way).

Why Are LTP and LTD Important?

They are how your brain adapts and rewires itself – ie neuroplasticity.

It's how:
- A child learns to ride a bike.
- A student remembers facts for an exam.
- A person can unlearn a fear or a bad habit.

In summary, Long-term potentiation (LTP) and long-term depression (LTD) are essential processes in neuroplasticity They enhance or reduce synaptic strength based on the frequency and pattern of stimulation (Citri & Malenka, 2008). These processes are fundamental for learning and memory.

CHAPTER 3

•———————•———————•

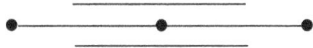

Neurogenesis or Creation of New Brain Cells

A remarkable part of Neuroplasticity is called Neurogenesis, which is worth spending some time on

Neurogenesis is the brain's process of creating new nerve cells, also known as neurons.

While many people think all our brain cells are made before we're born, children and teenagers continue to grow new nerve cells, especially in the parts of the brain that handle learning, memory, and emotions well into the mid-20s.

Where Does Neurogenesis Happen?

In children and teens, new nerve cells are mainly made in the Emotional circuits in the brain.

Let's start with the Mood and Memory Centre of the Brain (the Hippocampus). This mood and memory centre is found in the middle of the brain and is shaped like a seahorse.

It is a part of the brain that is crucial for:

• Learning and memory.
• Managing emotions.

There are other parts of the Emotional Circuitry of the brain like the Centre for Emotional Regulation (The Prefrontal Cortex), the Centre responsible for error detection and decision-making (The Angulate Cingulate Cortex) that also expands, ie gets more nerve cells in response to certain stimuli such as Physical Activity.

Why Is Neurogenesis Important in Childhood and Adolescence?

Because children's and teenagers' brains are still growing and wiring up, neurogenesis plays a huge role in how they learn, remember, and emotionally develop.

It helps them:
- Learn from experiences.
- Adapt to new situations.
- Regulate their emotions.
- Deal with challenges.

It is also one of the reasons children are so resilient – their brains are naturally more flexible and ready to change and grow.

What Helps Neurogenesis?

There are simple, natural ways to support healthy brain growth in children and teens:

Physical Activity
- Exercise (like running, swimming, dancing, playing football and countless others performed regularly) is one of the most powerful boosters of neurogenesis.

- It increases two hormones in the brain called Brain Derived Neurotrophic Factor (BNDF) and Insulin Like Growth Factor 1 (ILGF1) that act like "fertiliser" for growing new neurons (I'll expand on this later).

Good Sleep

I am going to devote a whole chapter to sleep as it is so massively important for all human beings, but a quick synopsis in the meantime:

- Deep sleep helps the brain clean out waste and strengthen new connections.
- Children who sleep well tend to remember more and regulate emotions better.

Healthy Nutrition

- A balanced diet with omega-3 fatty acids, nuts (if not allergic), fruits, vegetables, and protein fuels brain cell growth.

Loving Relationships

- Feeling safe and supported by parents and caregivers lowers stress and boosts brain development.
- Positive interactions actually help shape the brain's structure.

Low Stress

- Chronic stress can slow down neurogenesis, especially in the Emotional Control Centres.
- Helping kids manage stress with routines, mindfulness, and calm spaces protects their growing brains.

Now I know it is easy to say that all parents should provide children with a low stress environment. Of course, given the reality of life with all its twists and turns and trials and tribulations, it might be quite different.

Despite that, it is still worth knowing the mechanisms by which stress causes problems to and in the brain and how trying one's best to deal with your child's stress will potentially go a long way in reducing symptoms and facilitate recovery.

What Gets in the Way of Neurogenesis?

Certain things can interfere with healthy brain cell growth in children:
- Chronic stress or trauma.
- Neglect or social isolation.
- Poor sleep or nutrition.
- Lack of stimulation or learning due to excessive exposure to screens (smartphones and devices) which only provide passive stimulation.
- Lack of Physical Activity.

Fortunately, the young brain is incredibly adaptable. Even if a child has had a difficult start, the brain can still catch up with the right support.

I think to complete the picture of neuroplasticity for you it is worth focussing on how nerve cells communicate with each other: Brain wiring.

Brain wiring: for the 100 billion nerve cells in the brain to communicate effectively with each other they need to be connected by wiring.

This wiring is provided by Myelination and White Matter Maturation.

What Is Myelination?

Your child's brain is made up of billions of neurons – tiny nerve cells that send messages back and forth to control everything from walking to reading to emotions.

To work quickly and efficiently, these brain cells need insulation. That's what myelination is.

Myelination is the process where each neuron is wrapped in a fatty coating called myelin, like rubber insulation around an electrical wire. This helps messages travel faster and more reliably through the brain.

A very simple analogy to understand what myelin does is to think of a nerve cell without myelin like a road with multiple potholes, which makes driving heavy going and inefficient, not to mention how bad it can be on the tyres.

On the other hand, a myelinated neuron is like a motorway where traffic is flowing smoothly, meaning signals between nerve cells travel rapidly. The M25 by that analogy clearly has a deficiency of myelin.

What Is White Matter?

White matter is made up of all the myelinated connections in the brain. It links different parts of the brain together – like a superhighway system connecting cities.

The more mature and well-myelinated the white matter is, the faster and more efficiently your child's brain can think, learn, and regulate emotions.

When Does Myelination Happen?

Myelination starts before birth, but it continues all the way through childhood, adolescence, and even into the mid-20s!

The human brain's "wiring" is still developing for many years until the late teens, and because of that reason your child or teen may:

- Be impulsive or emotional (Emotional Control Centre not fully wired yet).
- Need repetition and practice to build strong brain pathways.
- Struggle with focus, organisation, or emotional regulation – especially in times of stress or growth.

This isn't a failure – it's normal brain development, and yes, whilst this behaviour can be very testing, please try to remember that your child or teenager is working at a disadvantage because the control systems necessary for mature behaviour are still immature.

Easier said than done, I know, but being aware of this and the fact that the behaviour is literally a phase might help you.

In addition, at a similar age your brain was going through the same transition. Speak to your parents and I am sure they will confirm that!

How Can Parents Support White Matter Maturation?

You can help your child's brain grow strong and efficient by supporting healthy myelination:

Physical Activity
- Regular movement and play boosts brain connectivity.
- Active children show stronger white matter and better learning skills.

Quality Sleep
- Myelination increases during deep sleep.
- Children need consistent sleep to consolidate learning and repair brain cells.

Learning and Practice
- Repetition and challenge (eg reading, puzzles, music, sports) strengthen neural wiring.
- The more a child uses a skill, the thicker the myelin around those brain pathways becomes.

Healthy Diet
- Fats like omega-3s (in fish), proteins, pulses, legumes, flaxseed, nuts (provided there are no allergies) are crucial for building myelin.
- Balanced nutrition supports brain development at every stage.
- Loving Relationships
- Secure attachment and low stress help the brain focus on growth, not survival.
- Chronic stress can disrupt myelination and slow down development.

Common Behavioural Manifestations linked with brain development and maturation.

Behaviour	Brain Explanation
Emotional outbursts	Prefrontal cortex still myelinating
Forgetfulness or disorganisation	Frontal white matter still under construction
Learning delays or processing speed issues	Immature white matter pathways
Impulsivity in teens	Myelination not complete until ~25 years

Final Takeaway:
The take home message is that providing your child with simple, inexpensive physical activities and trying to maintain as stable a home environment as possible will facilitate the healthy growth of your child's developing brain.

CHAPTER 4

• —— • —— •

Experience-Dependent Neuroplasticity

As brain plasticity is such a massively important part of human brain development and a topic of such huge significance as well as the premise of my book, I am going to dwell on it a bit longer with a few salient examples which are different from Physical Activity in order to convince you as to how multifaceted and remedial Brain Neuroplasticity can be.

This will hopefully help change the narrative that is traditionally assumed – once the brain is affected by illness or injury, not much can be done apart from treatment with medication and physiotherapy.

There is now incontrovertible evidence that neuroplasticity and life outcomes in children is heavily influenced by experience in life:

Enriched Environments

Evidence: Children raised in stimulating environments with social interaction, physical activity, and learning opportunities demonstrate superior cognitive, emotional, and nerve cell development (Greenough et al 1987).

Just imagine: the above seminal study was published nearly forty years ago but sadly seems to have been forgotten.

And even if it did generate interest back then, the message has long been forgotten, as a significant minority of parents who are unaware of the toxic effects of screens on children and teenagers have allowed technology such as smartphones, devices and social media apps to run their households rather than running the households themselves.

Animal studies show that enriched environments increase neuronal (nerve) branching, synaptic (junctions between nerves) density, and an increase in the number of nerve cells in the outer layer of the brain: the cortex.

Language Acquisition

The Language Centres of the Brain

The language centre in the brain is located mostly in the left side of the brain, especially in right-handed individuals.

Due to the amazing features of neuroplasticity, even if the left half of the brain is damaged, other areas (including the right hemisphere) can take over the language function, especially if damage occurs early.

Language development is a quintessential example of experience-dependent plasticity. Exposure to spoken language in early life is essential for development of vocabulary. Children deprived of language input (eg due to deafness or social neglect or excessive screen time) during critical periods may struggle to achieve full language.

Bilingualism (Learning two or more languages)

Children exposed to more than one language from an early age exhibit enhanced brain functioning and working memory.

Evidence: Bilingualism alters the structure of regions like the Emotional Control Centre (Prefrontal cortex), reflecting the brain's adaptation to increased stimulation from learning two languages (Green and Abutalebi 2013).

This fact alone does provide a very powerful reason for schools to make learning a second language compulsory.

Critical Period for Language Learning

The ability to acquire language peaks in early childhood, especially before the age of five. After puberty, learning a language requires more effort. It typically results in less fluency but due to its brain stimulating effects it is still very worthwhile.

In fact, science is now awash with studies proving that learning a second language can also help stave off dementia.

Other real-life manifestations of Neuroplasticity

Stroke and Brain Injury in Children

Unlike adults, children can often recover significant function after brain injuries due to their brain's plasticity.

Evidence: children who undergo removal of one cerebral hemisphere may still develop near-normal language and motor functions, particularly if the surgery occurs before age five (Helmstaedter et al 2003).

Autism Spectrum Disorder (ASD)

I have devoted a whole chapter to this later on.

Cerebral Palsy

Neuroplasticity offers a path for rehabilitation in cerebral palsy.

Evidence: Regular consistent movement therapy forces use of the affected limb and promotes reorganisation in the motor cortex which is the part of the brain controlling movement (Taub et al 2004).

Education and Learning

The understanding that learning physically changes the brain has inspired educational practices backed by research. The key strategies include the following:

Treatment of Learning Disabilities
Children with dyslexia show altered activity in the left side of the brain.

Evidence: Intensive phonological training can normalise brain activity and improve reading skills, illustrating the brain's capacity to rewire in response to targeted and repetitive stimulation (Shaywitz et al 2004).

Music Training
Learning to play an instrument boosts hearing and motor regions of the brain.

Evidence: Early music education is associated with improved verbal communication and memory (Hyde et al 2009).

So, learning a musical instrument doesn't just serve the purpose of embellishing the personal statement needed to apply to university! It is also hugely beneficial to promote growths of different parts of the brain and also helps prevent dementia later on in life.

Mindfulness and Meditation
Mindfulness training improves attention and emotional regulation.

Evidence: Brain scans show changes in the emotional control centres in the brain in children who engage in regular mindfulness practices (Zeidan et al 2010).

Adverse Experiences and Neuroplasticity

Trauma and Toxic Stress
Adverse Childhood Experiences can lead to maladaptive neuroplasticity or shrinkage of emotional centres in the brain in children.

Evidence: Chronic stress such as anxiety and depression alters the structure of various parts of the brain that have a crucial role in emotional well-being such as the Prefrontal cortex and Hippocampus (McEwen,

2000). These changes can impair emotional regulation, memory, and impulse control.

This will be explored in more detail in the relevant chapter.

Institutionalisation and Neglect

The heart wrenching stories of Romanian orphans and studies of children raised in Romanian orphanages show that prolonged deprivation leads to reduced brain size and cognitive deficits.

Evidence: Adoption into nurturing environments can partly reverse some of these effects, especially if it occurs before age two (Nelson et al 2007).

Real life implications

Neuroplasticity provides hope and a robust scientific basis for regular ongoing interventions tailored to the specific needs of the child or teenager. This is backed by the knowledge that considerable good and change can be achieved in the management of mental health disorders in children, teenagers and young adults by adopting simple changes to lifestyle such as physical activity and from a better understanding of how your child's brain works and what actions and approaches can facilitate healing.

There is definite and tangible hope based on the scientific fact of Neuroplasticty that Movement is Medicine.

CHAPTER 5

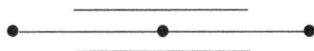

Changes in the brain due to anxiety and depression

In this chapter I am going to talk about Anxiety and Depression in Children and Teenagers, and spend some time on physical differences and neurochemical (chemical messenger) abnormalities in the brain leading into the next chapter which will discuss the Effectiveness of Physical activity in reversing some or all of these abnormalities.

It is now well established that anxiety and depression has sky-rocketed in the last 15 years amongst children and adolescents.

As per NHS England statistics published in late 2023, 20% (one in five) 8-25 year olds had a mental health disorder.

As anxiety and depression is now so common, if your child is struggling with anxiety or depression, you may wonder what's really going on in their brain.

These conditions are not just emotional problems, but underpinning these emotional problems are real, physical changes in how the brain functions, which is why it is worthwhile spending some time on this subject.

The good news is that the brain is still growing and changing during childhood and adolescence, and thanks to Neuroplasticity (that I have already discussed), many of these brain changes can improve over time.

This chapter explains what these brain differences are in a way that's easy to understand.

I am going to outline the brain's emotional control centres and emotional circuitry, and how these areas of the brain are affected in Anxiety and Depression:

The Brain's Alarm System (The Amygdala)

The Amygdala is located deep in the middle of the brain.

It is responsible for the following:
- Detects danger and triggers fear or stress.
- Helps your child react quickly when something feels threatening.

What are the key differences in anxiety and depression?
In children with anxiety, the amygdala is often more reactive; in other words, it gets set off or activated a bit too quickly, even when your child isn't in real danger.

In depression, it may overreact to sadness or social rejection.

How does this manifest?
- Constant worry, fear of new situations, panic attacks.
- Overreacting emotionally to small problems.
- Avoiding school or social situations because of fear.

The Centre for Emotional Regulation (Prefrontal Cortex)

This is the part of the brain right behind the forehead), it is *The Thinking and Calming Centre.*

What it does:
- Controls planning, decision-making, and managing emotions.
- Helps your child pause before reacting and think things through.

What's different:
- As mentioned previously, the prefrontal cortex is still developing in all children, but with anxiety and depression, it may be less active or develop more slowly.
- It also has trouble calming down the overactive brain's alarm system (the amygdala) as these two parts of the brain work very closely together.

What are the symptoms:
- Trouble focusing or making decisions.
- Difficulty calming down when upset.
- Feeling overwhelmed easily.

The Mood and Memory Centre (the Hippocampus)

This is located right next to the amygdala buried in the brain. It is shaped like a seahorse.

What it does:
- Stores memories and helps regulate emotions.
- Helps put things in context ("Is this really dangerous?").

What's different:
- In children with chronic stress or depression, the Hippocampus may be smaller or develop more slowly.
- *If a normal part of the brain shrinks, it means there is a loss of nerve cells and as a result, that part of the brain doesn't function as well as it should.*

What are the symptoms:
- Trouble remembering things.
- Getting stuck in negative memories.
- Holding onto sadness or fear from the past.

The Emotional Filter (Anterior Cingulate Cortex ACC)

This is also located at the front of the brain and looks like a collar.

Its function:
- Helps your child recognise and manage emotions.

What's different:
- May be underactive in children with depression, leading to difficulty processing feelings.
- May be overactive in anxiety, making it harder to stop worrying.

What this looks like:
- Constant overthinking or worrying.
- Not being able to "snap out" of a sad or anxious mood.

White Matter Pathways - The Brain's Communication Wires

What they do:
- Connect different brain regions so they can work seamlessly together.

What's different:
- In anxiety and depression, white matter development may be delayed and/or white matter might malfunction, ie send signals around the brain more slowly than normal.

- The brain's communication system is less efficient, especially between the various parts of the brain that make up the emotional circuitry.

What this looks like:
- Slower thinking or reaction time.
- Mood changes that seem sudden or hard to explain.

Thanks to neuroplasticity, children's brains are incredibly flexible. With love, support, and the right treatment – which must include physical activity – your child's brain can:
- Strengthen the thinking areas (prefrontal cortex).
- Calm the alarm system (amygdala).
- Build better communication pathways (white matter).
- Grow new brain cells in the Mood and Memory Centre (the Hippocampus) through activities like exercise and learning).

More on this with evidence in the next chapter

I have described a few parts of the brain that are responsible for the emotional circuitry. However, to complete the picture, I thought I would spend some time explaining the vital chemical messengers that are responsible for getting messages across nerve cells.

So what Are Neurochemicals?

Your child's brain communicates using neurochemicals – tiny messenger molecules that help brain cells, ie the nerve cells or neurons, "talk" to each other.

As you can imagine for such an incredibly mind boggling and complex organ like the brain to function properly, these neurochemicals must be present in optimum quantities to help transmit impulses between nerves seamlessly.

Some of the most important neurochemicals for emotions and mood include:

- Serotonin – helps regulate mood, sleep, and anxiety.
- Dopamine – linked to motivation, pleasure, and focus.
- Norepinephrine – involved in alertness and the stress response.
- GABA (gamma-aminobutyric acid) – helps calm the brain.
- Cortisol – a stress hormone that affects mood and energy.

When your child's brain has the right balance of these chemicals, it can manage emotions well. However, in anxiety and depression, this balance is often disrupted.

Neurochemical Imbalances in Anxiety and Depression

Serotonin – The Mood Stabiliser

- In depression: Serotonin levels are often too low, making it hard for the brain to feel calm or content.
- In anxiety: Low serotonin can make the brain more sensitive to threats and worry.

What it might look like:

- Sadness, irritability, panic, or emotional outbursts.
- Sleep problems or appetite changes.
- Feeling "on edge" or always worried.

Dopamine – The Motivation and Reward Chemical

- In depression, dopamine may be low, making it hard to feel joy or motivation.
- In anxiety, it may fluctuate, leading to restlessness or overthinking.

What it might look like:

- Lack of interest in favourite activities.
- Trouble starting or finishing tasks.
- Low energy or emotional "numbness".

Norepinephrine – The Alertness and Stress Responder

- Too much norepinephrine = anxiety and panic.
- Too little = fatigue and low mood.

What it might look like:

- Jumpy, easily startled, constant "what if" thoughts.
- Tired but unable to relax or sleep.
- Mood swings and irritability.

Gamma Aminobutyric Acid GABA – The Calming Chemical

- In anxiety, GABA may be too low, so the brain can't slow down or "turn off" worrying thoughts.

What it might look like:

- Trouble falling asleep or relaxing.
- Overreacting to small problems.
- Needing constant reassurance.

Cortisol – The Stress Hormone

- Cortisol is released when your child is under stress.

- In children with chronic anxiety or depression, cortisol stays high for too long and can affect the brain's ability to regulate emotions.

What it might look like:
- Tiredness, trouble concentrating.
- Physical symptoms (headaches, stomach aches).
- Emotional meltdowns or shutting down.

Why Do These Imbalances Happen?
Neurochemical problems in anxiety and depression can be caused by:
- Genetics – some children are born with more sensitive brain chemistry.
- Stress or trauma – bullying, family conflict, or big life changes can change brain chemicals.
- Sleep problems – poor sleep affects serotonin and dopamine levels.
- Lack of physical activity and or healthy nutrition – the brain needs physical activity and healthy food to make the right chemicals.
- Loneliness or isolation – social connection boosts feel-good brain chemicals like oxytocin which will be discussed later.

The beauty about knowing the intricacies of the brain's structure and workings through neurochemicals is that it provides us with the ability to optimise the functioning of these essential components of brain function – which leads me nicely on to the next chapter.

CHAPTER 6

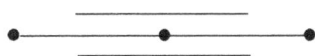

Physical Activity (PA) as a treatment for Anxiety and Depression in Children and Teenagers

What does the science tell us about the medicinal or therapeutic effects of physical activity on the brain?

For me to convince you of these facts and give you confidence that PA can be very beneficial for the brain, we will need to take a bit of a deep dive into how physical activity works backed by evidence.

Physical changes in the brain following physical activity:

The Communication Pathways of the Brain (White Matter)

Regular physical activity significantly improves the structure of white matter, the brain's communication highways.

Evidence: A study of seven- to nine-year-olds showed that a nine-month after-school fitness programme enhanced white matter structure, ie communication between brain cells was better (Chaddock-Heyman et al 2018).

Faster, better connected brains help children regulate emotions, focus more easily, and process information more smoothly, skills often impaired by anxiety and depression.

The Mood and memory Centre (The Hippocampus)

The Hippocampus is frequently smaller, ie, it has shrunk in youth with depression, which in turn has an impact on the child's mood and memory.

Evidence: Several studies have demonstrated that regular aerobic exercise such as playing football, cycling, swimming and running etc can lead to an increase in the number of nerve cells in the Mood and Memory Centre, which leads to an improvement in depressive symptoms.

Evidence: Exercise training increases size of hippocampus and improves memory (Kirk I Erickson, Michelle W Voss et al 2011).

Strengthening Emotion Control Centres: (The Prefrontal Cortex (PFC) and Anterior Cingulate Cortex (ACC))

Exercise leads to an increased number of nerve cells and optimum functioning in the regions essential for emotion regulation and executive functioning.

Evidence: A six-month brisk walking routine resulted in increased number of nerve cells in the PFC and ACC (Colcombe et al 2006).

Another study using highly sensitive and accurate MRI brain scans to study the effects of exercise on the brain concluded that physical activity during childhood may improve brain function involved in attention, working memory, and decision-making (cognition) (Chadoock Heyman et al 2013).

Body's Stress Response System (Hypothalamic-Pituitary-Adrenal HPA axis).

The HPA axis is a very important part of your child's stress response system like an internal alarm system that helps the body deal with stress or danger by:

- Increasing heart rate.
- Raising blood sugar (for quick energy).
- Sharpening focus.

This is often called the "fight or flight" response.

If a child experiences long-term stress, like family problems, bullying, or anxiety, the HPA axis can stay switched on too much of the time leading to high levels of the stress hormone cortisol. This may in turn lead to:

- Difficulty sleeping.
- Mood changes.
- Trouble focusing.
- Shrinkage of the Mood and Memory Centre (The Hippocampus).

Evidence: Exercise, particularly aerobic exercise such as football, cycling and running etc, can lead to reduced activation of the body's stress response system, leading to a more balanced stress hormone (cortisol) secretion (Rodriguez et al 2024).

Intensity Helps:

Exercise intensity plays a role, with moderate to vigorous intensity exercise often showing a greater impact on stress hormone (cortisol) levels compared to lower intensity activities. Playing football or any team sport is a great stress buster (A Caplin et al 2021).

Consistent exercise habits, even if moderate, can have positive, long-term effects on the HPA axis and the child is better able to deal with the various stresses of life.

Neurochemicals:

Traditionally the first line of treatment for the vast majority of mental health disorders is medication.

These drugs work by increasing the levels of the essential neurochemicals in the brain that I have already listed and have spent quite a lot of time discussing.

These drugs can be effective; however, they need to be taken for long periods of time, and often have side effects. In addition, coming off these medicines can be quite difficult

But guess what! Physical activity works in pretty much the same way, ie by normalising depleted neurochemicals but also increasing the levels of certain hormones that promote the growth of nerve cells.

Below is a narrative of the various hormones and chemicals that are increased by physical activity:

Nerve Growth Hormone: Brain-Derived Neurotrophic Factor (BDNF)

BDNF is a critical hormone that supports nerve cell growth, like a fertiliser for young brains.

Evidence: Moderate to high intensity aerobic exercise, such as running, swimming or cycling etc, results in an increase in the nerve growth hormone levels in children and young people (de Menzes – Junior et al 2022).

The resulting increase in BDNF levels following exercise are associated with improvements in memory, attention and executive functions of which are all vital for academic and daily life performance.

IGF-1 (Insulin-like Growth Factor 1) is a hormone with a structure similar to insulin.

IGF-1 is critically important for brain development, function, repair, and plasticity, ie it is another fertiliser for the brain.

In addition, it improves levels of dopamine and serotonin which affect mood and motivation.

And the 'pièce de résistance' is below.

Physical activity increases both BDNF and IGF-1, enhancing cognitive performance and mental health, especially in children and adolescents.

Evidence: In adolescent schoolchildren, an eight-week treadmill programme (three times per week) significantly increased both blood IGF1 and BDNF, suggesting that aerobic workouts boost nerve growth hormone levels during brain development (Kyun Jeon et al 2015).

Serotonin: The Mood Stabiliser whose levels are usually reduced in anxiety and depression

Exercise increases serotonin levels, which are usually depleted in depression.

Evidence: Physical activity like running, jumping, and playing team sports like basketball etc elevates serotonin, improving mood and reducing depressive symptoms (Teymori et al 2019).

Team sport, group activities and outdoor play are particularly beneficial.

Dopamine levels linked to motivation, pleasure and focus, which are depressed in Anxiety and Depression, are optimised by exercise.

Evidence: Aerobic exercise like cycling increases the release of dopamine, the neurotransmitter associated with motivation, reward, and mood regulation (Gorrell et al 2022).

Endorphins

What Are Endorphins?
Endorphins are chemicals which are so called because they are block pain and produce feelings of well-being.

Reduce Stress and Anxiety
- Endorphins calm the brain by blocking stress signals.
- Endorphins are released during laughter, physical touch, teamwork, and shared fun.
- This helps children feel more connected to others and builds social confidence and in turn stronger relationships, reduced loneliness, and better peer support.
- *Evidence:* Running led to measurable increases in the body's endorphin levels as measured in a group of runners (Boecker et el 2008).

Lowering Cortisol

Exercise helps regulate the stress hormone cortisol, preventing chronic elevation that damages the brain and sustains mood disorders.

Evidence for Reduced Cortisol Levels
Studies have shown that children with higher levels of physical activity exhibit a reduced increase in cortisol levels in response to stress.

Evidence: **active children had minimal or no increase in cortisol** in response to stress, while children in lower physical activity groups had **significant cortisol spikes (Martikainen et al 2013).**

Gamma Amino Butyric Acid (GABA) calms brain activity, reduces stress, and helps regulate mood, attention, and sleep.

Physical activity stimulates GABA synthesis in the brain, particularly in Emotional Control Centres.

Evidence: Aerobic exercise boosts GABA and can be as effective as medication in reducing mild to moderate anxiety and depression (Coxon et al in 2018).

In case you are still not convinced about the evidence, I thought I would share two more studies with you.

One a pretty large study and the other one a massive study, in fact probably one of the biggest ever done.

- 1. A Swedish study conducted over a period of four years in 16,000 youths, showed that each extra hour of activity at age 11 reduced psychiatric diagnosis risk by 12%, anxiety by 40%, and depression by 25%.
- 2. A large Taiwanese study of two million children aged 10–11 found that higher fitness levels correlated with lower anxiety and depression rates and improvements in ADHD symptoms.

Bringing It Together

There have been hundreds of research trials examining the effects of physical activity (PA) on depression, anxiety and psychological distress.

Many of these studies suggest that PA may have similar effects to psychotherapy and treatment with medication (and with numerous advantages over psychotherapy and pharmacotherapy, in terms of cost, side-effects and associated health benefits).

All modes of PA were effective, and higher intensity exercise was associated with even greater improvements for depression and anxiety.

What you should do:

Encourage at least 30-45 minutes of moderate activity, like running, dancing, cycling, or playing team sports etc – three or more times a week.

Why it matters:
You're not just helping your child stay active – you're literally rewiring their brain to be more resilient, happier, and focused.

What you will see:
Better mood, reduced worry, improved concentration, more energy, and emotional stability.

Long-term pay off:
Supporting mental health naturally, reducing reliance on medications, and laying a foundation for lifelong brain health.

CHAPTER 7

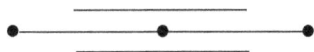

Brain changes in ADHD and Tech ADHD

ADHD (Attention-Deficit Hyperactivity Disorder) is a condition that affects how a child thinks, feels, and acts.

The incidence is seven per 100 children, although the number of children, teenagers and adults being diagnosed is increasing dramatically for a variety of reasons.

At the outset, it is worth stating that ADHD is not caused by poor parenting, laziness or a lack of discipline; indeed, children with ADHD have measurable differences in how their brains are structured and how they function.

I am going to set out some of these differences below.

The Brain Develops More Slowly in Some Areas

- In children with ADHD, some brain areas develop more slowly than in other children.
- These delays are often seen in the Centre for Emotional Regulation (the Prefrontal Cortex) – the part of the brain responsible for attention, planning, impulse control, and organisation.
- On average, this part of the brain matures two to three years later in children with ADHD.

What this looks like: A child may have difficulty sitting still, staying focused, or remembering instructions – not because they aren't trying, but because their brain is still catching up in these areas.

Differences in Brain Size and Structure

- Very sensitive and accurate brain scans show that some areas of the brain are slightly smaller in children with ADHD, especially:
  - Centre for Emotional Regulation (Prefrontal cortex) just behind the forehead that controls attention and decision-making).
  - The Motivation and Movement Centre (Basal ganglia nerve cells found deep within the brain).
  - The Movement and Balance Centre (Cerebellum located at the back of the brain which also plays a role in emotional control).

These size differences are consistent across studies and the fact that they are smaller is because these parts of the brain have less nerve cells than normal.

What this means: These physical differences can make it harder for children with ADHD to control impulses, manage their emotions, or shift focus between tasks.

Reduced Communication Between Brain Regions

The brain consists of bundles of nerve fibres called white matter that connect different regions of the brain, allowing for fast communication between areas responsible for attention, impulse control, planning, and emotional regulation.

In ADHD, the structure of the white matter is not normal, which can lead to problems with emotional regulation.

Lower Levels of Key Brain Chemicals (Neurotransmitters)

Children with ADHD often have lower levels of dopamine and serotonin, two brain chemicals that help with:

- Attention.
- Motivation.
- Reward and pleasure.

These chemicals help messages travel between brain cells. When levels are low or not balanced, the brain has trouble keeping thoughts and actions on track; it is literally like having a patchy internet signal.

What this means: Children with ADHD may need more stimulation or feedback to stay engaged.

The brain responds differently to rewards and consequences.

Brain imaging studies (fMRI, PET) reveal altered activity in the brain's "motivation and reward circuit".

As a result, these children may:

- Find it harder to stay motivated by long-term goals.
- React strongly to immediate, exciting rewards, but struggle with tasks that don't give instant feedback.
- Example: A sticker at the end of the day may not be as motivating as praise or a reward given immediately after a task.

Important Things to Remember

- ADHD is not a child's fault nor is it the parents' fault.
- It's a neurological difference, ie children with ADHD have brains that are wired differently and are often maturing more slowly.

TECH ADHD

At this point I would like to introduce a relatively new concept, a condition called Tech Induced ADHD or Acquired ADHD.

When children spend excessive time on screens – especially on fast-paced, highly stimulating platforms like TikTok, YouTube Shorts, Instagram, or video games – their brains can become wired to seek constant stimulation.

This can lead to attention problems that *look* like ADHD.

This is sometimes called "tech-induced ADHD" or Acquired ADHD", because the symptoms mimic real ADHD, but the root cause is behavioural and environmental, not neurological or genetic.

Symptoms You Might Notice

The child might:
- Struggle to focus on homework, reading, or conversations.
- Seem bored or restless when not on a screen.
- Jump quickly between tasks or apps.
- Become irritable or anxious when screens are taken away.
- Have disrupted sleep, poor memory, or impulsivity.

These behaviours can resemble inattentive or hyperactive ADHD, but they often started after screen habits worsened.

Why Does This Happen?

Apps and games are designed to be addictive by:
- Delivering instant gratification (likes, videos, rewards).

- Releasing dopamine, a brain chemical linked to pleasure and motivation.
- Shortening attention spans by rewarding quick shifts in focus.

Over time, this reconditions the brain to expect stimulation at all times, making slower tasks – like reading, listening in class, or doing chores – feel boring or frustrating.

Evidence: In a recent study the researching team tracked teenagers who spent many hours per day on social media over a period of a couple of years and a separate group of teenagers who were more disciplined with screen use.

When these teenagers were assessed at the end of the study, they found that those teenagers who spent many hours each and every week on smartphones and social media developed symptoms such as hyperactivity, inattention impulsivity and poor sleep (Chaelin K. Ra et al 2018).

The reason for this is that excessive screen and social media app time causes structural changes and dysfunction in the areas of the brain that we have already discussed which are responsible for emotional regulation.

Tech ADHD or Acquired ADHD can even affect preschool children who spend long periods of time on devices.

This Acquired ADHD is likely to be contributing substantially to the increased diagnosis of children with ADHD, although unlike children with Primary ADHD, the behavioural manifestations are due to brain changes secondary to excessive smartphone, device and social media app use.

The important take home message is that screen-induced attention problems are learned behaviours and usually improve with lifestyle changes, ie moderating and controlling excessive screen use.

The other really important lesson that science is telling us is that allowing a child with Primary ADHD to have too much screen time could potentially be making the underlying ADHD worse.

The reason for that is that excessive screen time leads to changes in the Emotional Control centres of the brain which are already affected in Primary ADHD, thereby potentially making matters worse.

What Can Parents Do?

1. Lead by example
Not that you need evidence as this next statement is so obvious, but for the disbelievers, there is actually plenty of evidence that children copy their parents and using tech is no different.

2. Set Healthy Boundaries
- Limit daily recreational screen time which is governed by a child's age.
- Use screen-free zones (like bedrooms, dinner tables, outings etc).
- Create consistent tech routines (on/off times, no screens before bed).

3. Encourage Real-World Activities, More Green Time, Less Screen Time
- Sports, creative hobbies, outdoor time, reading.
- Play-based learning for younger kids.
- More Green Time less Screen Time.

Movement is Medicine: Physical Activity as a treatment for ADHD is explored in more detail in the next chapter.

CHAPTER 8

Physical Activity for ADHD

In this chapter I am going to focus on Physical Activity (PA) as a treatment for ADHD (Attention Deficit Hyperactivity Disorder) and to explain the mechanisms by which physical activity, by addressing the various clinical manifestations of ADHD, can help minimise the use of medication in these children.

Studies show that physical activity can improve motor skills, executive functions (planning and organising), and reduce symptoms like anxiety, depression, and aggressive behaviour. It can also lead to better mood, increased energy, and a boost in serotonin and dopamine in the brain which is exactly how the ADHD medicines work.

Changes in the physical structure of the brains in children with ADHD as a result of Physical Activity:
- The Centre for Emotional Regulation (The Prefrontal Cortex) is responsible for attention, planning, impulse control, **and** working memory – all areas that are impaired in ADHD.
- Physical activity increases blood flow, oxygen delivery, and BDNF (Brain-Derived Neurotrophic Factor), the hormone that leads to growth of neurons in this region.

Evidence: An overview of a number of research studies of ADHD youth found that physical activity had moderate-to-large effects in terms of improved attention span, better focus, and greater self-regulation (Dong Li et al 2023).

Strengthening of White Matter Tracts which are the communication pathways between the brain cells

- Children with ADHD often have reduced white matter, which disrupts communication between brain regions.
- Exercise has been shown to improve white matter structure. *Evidence:* Children in a ninemonth aerobic programme showed stronger white matter compared with inactive peers (ChaddockHeyman et al 2018):
- Activities like aerobic exercise and coordination training help strengthen these tracts.

Result: Faster and more efficient brain communication and processing.

The Mood and Memory Centre (The Hippocampus)

- The hippocampus, involved in learning and memory, is often smaller in children with ADHD.
- Regular physical activity (especially aerobic such as running, cycling, swimming and of course football and other team sports) increases formation of new nerve cells in the hippocampus.
- This is partly due to increased nerve growth hormones BDNF and IGF1 which support nerve cell growth and blood vessel formation.

Result: Improved memory, learning, and emotional regulation.

Evidence: Overweight, sedentary children (7–11 yrs) joined a three-month aerobic after-school programme. Children in the high-exercise group (40 min/day) had improved hippocampal-dependent memory and greater activity in the hippocampus on MRI scans (Davis et al 2011).

The Cerebellum

The cerebellum (in coordination, balance and emotional regulation), is often smaller in children with ADHD.

Evidence: Exercise enhances cerebellar function and structure, improving motor control, balance and coordination (Y S Chan et al 2021)

Improved Executive Functions:
- Executive functions are brain skills like planning, organising, switching tasks, and remembering instructions and are often weaker in children with ADHD.
- Exercise boosts blood flow and brain plasticity, strengthening areas like the prefrontal cortex (responsible for executive function).
- Exercise, particularly aerobic exercise such as cycling, running or trampolining with appropriate safeguards can improve executive functions like attention, improve thinking, language, learning and memory.
- All of this can in turn lead to a reduction in core ADHD symptoms such as inattention, hyperactivity and impulsivity.
- *Evidence:* six weeks of daily morning exercise before school led to better task-switching, working memory, and self-control in primary school children with ADHD (Pontifex et al 2016).

Enhanced Neurotransmitters:
- Aerobic exercise like playing football, running, cycling, swimming etc increases levels of dopamine, serotonin and norepinephrine, key brain chemicals that are low in children with ADHD.

- These chemicals help with attention, concentration, and impulse control – just like ADHD medications do.

Evidence: Just 20 minutes of moderate-intensity exercise led to improved attention and reduced impulsivity in children with ADHD – effects similar to a low dose of stimulant medication such as Ritalin (Wigal et al 2013).

Even a brisk walk to school of about 20 minutes will have a positive effect.

For further benefits on the ADHD symptoms, challenging the body as well as the brain with complex activities like martial arts, ballet, ice skating, gymnastics, rock climbing, and mountain biking seem to have a greater positive impact on children with ADHD than aerobic exercise.

Martial arts, ie karate, is my go-to exercise as I have been a practitioner and proponent of Shotokan karate for nearly 40 years and I can vouch for its benefits.

Reduces Hyperactivity and Impulsivity

Children with ADHD often feel the need to move constantly. Giving them structured physical activity:

- Helps them burn off excess energy.
- Makes it easier to sit still and focus in the classroom afterwards.
- Reduces disruptive behaviour.

Evidence: A study carried out in 2020 concluded that school-based physical activity programmes led to measurable improvements in hyperactivity and impulse control in children with ADHD. Even short bursts of activity, like a 15-minute walk or game, can calm behaviour and improve classroom conduct in children with ADHD (Dong Li et al 2020).

Improves Mood and Reduces Anxiety
- Many children with ADHD also struggle with anxiety, low self-esteem, or mood swings.
- Physical activity increases GABA, serotonin, and endorphins – chemicals that calm the brain and improve mood.

Evidence: A review of the research evidence in *2022* found that regular physical activity significantly reduced anxiety and emotional distress in children with ADHD (Seiifer et al 2022).

Helps with Sleep
Many children with ADHD struggle with falling asleep, staying asleep, or waking up too early. Poor sleep can make ADHD symptoms worse – increasing hyperactivity, impulsivity, and trouble with focus.

Evidence: A *study by Smilt et al 2013* followed children with ADHD who took part in regular physical activity programmes over 12 weeks. The results showed the following key points:
- Faster time to fall asleep.
- Fewer nighttime awakenings.
- Better overall sleep quality.
- Improved daytime behaviour and attention.

"Physical activity may serve as a non-pharmaceutical approach to improving sleep and behaviour in children with ADHD," the researchers concluded.

However, I would caution against a child with ADHD undertaking vigorous physical activity just before bedtime as that is likely to be counterproductive.

Improves Academic Performance and Classroom Behaviour
Regular movement, especially before or during school outside of lessons of course, can:

- Increase focus during lessons.
- Reduce fidgeting and interruptions.
- Improve learning and memory.

Evidence: A study in 2016 found that children with ADHD who participated in a daily 30-minute physical activity programme showed significant improvements in attention, behaviour, and mood (Song et al).

What kind of exercise works best?

Type of Exercise	How It Helps
Aerobic (eg football, running swimming, biking)	Boosts brain chemicals (dopamine, norepinephrine)
Martial arts (eg karate, taekwondo)	Improves self-control, discipline, and body awareness
Team sports	Builds social skills and focus through structure
Yoga / mindfulness-based movement	Calms the nervous system, improves attention
Short movement breaks	Increases classroom focus and reduces restlessness

The most important factor to consider when starting an exercise programme is to find something that your child enjoys doing – at least that way your child will stick with it.

Furthermore, at least two studies have suggested that physical activity done in nature reduces ADHD symptoms significantly more than activities done in other settings.

Evidence:(Kuo, 2004 and Taylor, 2009) which chimes nicely with what I advise to parents and families: More Green Time Less Screen Time

In conclusion, in this chapter I have focused on how physical activity addresses the majority of the salient features of ADHD backed by sound science and I fervently hope that Physical Activity becomes an integral and routine part of the management of children and teenagers with ADHD.

CHAPTER 9

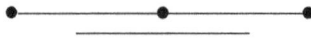

Brain changes in Autism

Autism Spectrum Disorder (ASD) is a developmental condition that affects how a child thinks, communicates, and interacts with the world around them.

Research using modern and accurate brain scans have shown that there are structural and neurochemical differences in the brains of children and teenagers with ASD compared to those without.

I have described these in order to help parents, children and families understand what the differences are, which will make caring for these children easier.

1. **Larger Brain Size in Early Childhood:** Many children with autism have larger brain sizes, in early life, particularly between ages two to four.

   As a result of this increase in the brain size, the nerve cells seem to struggle to connect with each other as well as they otherwise would.

   This helps us understand the reason why some autistic children show early language or social delays.

2. **Differences in the Bundle of Nerves connecting the two halves of the brain together (the Corpus Callosum)**
   In many children with autism, these connections are less well-developed which in turn may make it harder for the brain's two

sides to communicate efficiently and effectively, thereby affecting coordination, problem-solving, or emotional processing.

3. **Changes in the Brain's Alarm Centre (the Amygdala)** which helps us recognize emotions and respond to threats or social cues. In autism: the amygdala may be different in structure compared to other children, which could explain why autistic children have heightened anxiety, difficulty recognizing emotions in others, or being overwhelmed by too much stimulation.

4. **Changes in the Emotional Control Centres in the Brain:** Studies have indicated that children with autism spectrum disorder often exhibit abnormalities in the prefrontal cortex (PFC), particularly in nerve cell number and connectivity – this area is involved in planning, decision-making, and social behaviour.

5. **Temporal lobe:** located in the middle of the brain, is important for understanding language and recognizing faces.

    In autism: Both areas may show differences in size, shape, or connectivity.

    What this may affect: Children might struggle with social rules or understanding spoken language and facial expressions.

6. **Movement and Balance Centre (the Cerebellum)**, which is a structure at the back of the brain, is crucial for fine motor coordination, balance, precise timing of movements as well as emotional well-being.

    Research consistently points to a decrease in the size of the cerebellum in ASD and that may play a role in the diverse range of symptoms associated with the condition.

What This Means for children with ASD

- These brain differences do not mean a child with ASD is abnormal but that the autistic brain works in a different and unusual way.
- Many children with ASD develop new skills over time, especially with the right support.
- Early intervention, understanding, and patience make a huge difference in helping children with ASD thrive.

Neurochemical Differences in Children with Autism

Neurochemicals are the tiny chemical messengers that help brain cells "talk" to each other.

In children with autism, several key neurotransmitters seem to behave differently, which may help explain some of their unique behaviours, challenges and strengths.

1. GABA (Gamma-Aminobutyric Acid): The Calming Messenger

What it does: GABA is the brain's soothing balm" – it helps calm the brain and reduces anxiety and overstimulation. Research shows that children with ASD may have lower GABA activity.

How this might affect a child with ASD:

- May be more sensitive to noise, touch, or lights.
- Could have trouble calming down or regulating emotions.
- Might feel overwhelmed more easily.

2. Glutamate: The Exciting Messenger

What it does: Glutamate helps with learning, memory, and brain development.

In autism: Some children may have too much glutamate activity, or an imbalance between glutamate and GABA.

What this means:
- The brain might be overactive in certain areas.
- Can contribute to hyperactivity, anxiety, or repetitive behaviours.

Serotonin: The Mood and Sensory Messenger

What it does: Serotonin helps regulate mood, sleep, appetite, and sensory perception.

In autism: Around one-third of children with autism have abnormal levels of serotonin in their blood.

How it might affect a child with ASD:
- May be related to repetitive behaviours or rigid routines.
- Could influence sleep patterns or gut issues (since serotonin also affects digestion).

4. Dopamine: The Motivation and Reward Messenger
What it does: Dopamine helps with attention, motivation, reward, and movement.

In autism: Dopamine systems in the brain may be underactive in certain areas.

Impact on a child with ASD:
- Might affect attention, focus, and impulse control.
- Plays a role in social reward, ie why some autistic children may not find social interaction as rewarding as others.

5. Oxytocin: The Social Bonding Messenger

What it does: This hormone helps with social bonding, trust, and empathy, for instance, facilitating the emotional connection between parents and their children.

In autism: Some children may have lower oxytocin levels.

Possible effects:

- Might struggle with making eye contact or understanding others' feelings.
- May prefer being alone or have difficulty with group play.

I have outlined these differences in the brains of children with ASD to provide a better understanding whilst simultaneously offering hope based on the existence of neuroplasticity as to how these variations can be addressed with the help of Physical Activity in the next chapter.

CHAPTER 10

Physical Activity as a Treatment for ASD

Evidence that Physical Activity has a therapeutic effect in children with Autistic Spectrum Disorder (ASD).

The beauty about physical activity is that it is extremely beneficial for a very wide variety of mental health disorders in childhood and adolescence, regardless of the complexity.

Autistic Spectrum Disorder is one such complex condition which is very amenable to the wide ranging physical and neurochemical benefits of physical activity as set out below.

Improvements in Brain structure

Improved White Matter which are the brain's connecting pathways

Evidence: A 2021 study by Yang et al showed that structured physical activity (like aerobic games and movement-based play such as team sports or martial arts) improved connectivity between brain cells in children with ASD, particularly between regions involved in social, communication and motor control.

Why it matters:

Better white matter structure means better brain efficiency, which can help with communication, behaviour regulation, and adapting to changes.

Growth in the Mood and Memory Centre (the Hippocampus) and other parts of the Brain involved in Emotional Regulation

Evidence: A 2020 study by Den Ouden et al using MRI scans found that 12 weeks of aerobic exercise (cycling, swimming, running, team sports) led to increased volume in the hippocampus – a brain region involved in memory, emotional regulation, and learning – in children with developmental disorders, including ASD.

What this helps with:
- Memory and learning.
- Helping children feel more secure in routines.

Changes in the Cerebellum (involved in coordination, movement and emotions):

Children with ASD often have structural differences in the cerebellum

Evidence: Research from 2022 by Wan Chun Su et al using movement-based interventions (like balance training, martial arts, or yoga) showed positive changes in cerebellar activity and motor cortex function.

How it helps:
- Better balance and coordination.
- Greater confidence in physical and social activities.

Increased Growth Hormones and Neurochemicals after Physical Activity

Increased levels of Hormones responsible for growth of nerve cells: Brain-Derived Neurotrophic Factor (BDNF)

Evidence: Multiple studies have shown that physical activity increases levels of BDNF – a brain growth protein that supports the development of new brain cells and connections.

How it helps children with autism:

- Encourages neuroplasticity (the brain's ability to change and grow).
- Supports learning and social development.

Insulin-like Growth Factor 1 (IGF-1) is a hormone critical for brain development. It plays a role in:

- Myelination (the insulating layer of nerve cells in the brain).
- Growth of nerve cells.
- Synapse formation or increased connections between nerve cells.

Evidence: Kim et al 2016 studied school-aged children with autism who participated in eight weeks of structured physical activity (aerobic and coordination-based exercise).

Results: Significant improvements in social skills and cognitive scores, which the authors partially attributed to increased IGF-1 and BDNF levels in the blood.

These studies suggest that physical activity can promote nerve growth hormone production, leading to the creation of new nerve cells that results in improvements in symptoms in children with autism.

Physical Activity Boosts The Brain's "Calming Balm" Chemical (GABA)

Evidence: Coxon et al, 2017: High-intensity exercise raised GABA levels in the brain's emotional and movement centres by about 20%. GABA helps the brain slow down and regulate reactions.

Why it matters for autism:
- Helps with emotional regulation.
- Supports better focus and behaviour control.

The Brain's "Go" Signal (Glutamate)

What the evidence says:
In autism, glutamate levels are often too high, which may contribute to overstimulation or anxiety.

Evidence: Exercise has been shown to help rebalance glutamate (Maddock et al 2016).

Benefits for a child with ASD:
- May reduce repetitive movements or meltdowns.
- Helps the brain respond more flexibly to new situations.

Increases Dopamine – The Motivation and Focus Chemical

Aerobic activity (like football, running, swimming, or cycling etc) increases dopamine levels in the brain.

Evidence: Sansi et al 2019 Children with autism (ages 7–12) participated in a 12-week aerobic exercise programme (running and cycling).

Results: The children showed improved attention and focus.

Why this helps children with autism:
- Improves attention and reduces distractibility.
- Helps increase motivation and participation in tasks.

Raises Serotonin – The Mood and Sleep Stabiliser

Serotonin is often irregular in children with ASD. Physical activity has been shown to increase serotonin levels, which helps with mood, sleep, and sensory regulation.

Evidence: Cumulative empirical evidence demonstrated a substantial rise in serotonin levels after engaging in physical exercise (Alghadir et al 2016).

How it helps:
- Improved mood and reduced anxiety.
- Better sleep patterns.
- Fewer emotional outbursts or sensory-related distress.

Boosts Endorphins – The Brain's Natural "Feel-Good" Chemicals

What the evidence says:
Endorphins are released during moderate-to-vigorous physical activity. Children with autism often show improved mood and behaviour after exercise due to increased endorphin levels.

Evidence: Iversen et al 2020 Noted that physical activity induces endorphin release, supports emotion regulation and improved behavioural outcome.

How physical activity helps:
- Mood and emotional regulation.
- Reduction in stereotypic and repetitive behaviours.
- Lowered stress and anxiety levels.

Increases Oxytocin – The "Connection" Chemical
Oxytocin helps build social bonds, trust, and empathy.

How it helps:
- Supports social connection and eye contact.
- Reduces fear and improves emotional warmth.

Evidence: Tsukamoto et al 2024 showed a significant increase in oxytocin levels in young adults following intense exercise and even more gratifying for me, Yassovsky et al showed in 2019 that the practice of martial arts is associated with an increase in oxytocin levels.

These increased levels can lead to improved social responsiveness and reduced repetitive behaviours.

There are some studies that describe using this chemical as a medicine so why not increase the levels by encouraging a child with ASD to participate in regular physical activity?

Physical activity is much, much healthier, it is effective and has no side effects.

What Kind of Activities Work Best?

Whatever your child likes and will do regularly; however, a few common beneficial physical activities are listed below:

Aerobic exercises: swimming, biking, jumping on a trampoline.

Structured games: obstacle courses, tag, relay races.

Martial arts like karate, which I am partial to as a veteran student and practitioner of this martial art helps builds self-control and body awareness.

Social physical activities: dancing, team sports, or partner games.

Sensory play-based movement: swings, climbing, animal walks.

Frequency: Just 30–60 minutes a day, three times a week can make a huge difference and I have presented you with the science to back that up.

CHAPTER 11

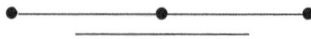

Physical changes in the Brain due to Excessive Screen time and Social media use: The SCREEN DEMIC

The human brain is still developing throughout childhood and into the mid-20s, especially in areas that control emotion, attention, and decision-making. Too much time spent on smartphones, devices and social media can disrupt this development in specific, measurable ways.

Social media is the ubiquitous and universally recognised term; however, given its addictive nature and toxic effects on the brain, it is often categorically antisocial.

Physical changes in the brain

1. **Changes in the Centre for Emotional Regulation (Prefrontal Cortex)**
   - The prefrontal cortex controls impulse control, planning, decision-making, and emotional regulation.
   - Excessive screen use is associated with delayed maturation and reduced nerve cells in this area.
   - Children may become more impulsive, less able to focus, and emotionally reactive.

2. **Disrupted Brain Connectivity (Impaired white matter pathways)**
   - Studies using very sensitive brain scans show that children who spend many hours on screens have less organised white matter in key brain pathways, especially in those areas of the brain responsible for language development and self-control.
   - Impaired white matter, which is responsible for connecting the brain cells or neurons with each other, results in slower processing speed and difficulties in communication and learning.

3. **Reward System Overactivation (Addiction-like Brain Patterns)**
   - Social media triggers frequent dopamine release – the brain's "feel-good" chemical – similar to what happens with gambling or substance use.
   - Over time, this can lead to overactive reward circuits, especially in two of the emotional control centres in the brain called the striatum and amygdala, which may cause:
     - Craving for likes and constant checking.
     - Mood swings and irritability when offline.
     - Reduced sensitivity to natural rewards (eg, family time or hobbies).

4. **Shrinking of the Centre for Focus and Empathy (Anterior Cingulate Cortex)**
   - Excessive screen time is linked with reduced nerve cells in the anterior cingulate cortex, which supports attention, empathy, and emotional awareness.
   - This may lead to:

- ○ Shorter attention spans.
- ○ Decreased empathy.
- ○ Poorer emotional self-awareness.

5. **Disruption of Sleep and Body Clock (Circadian) Rhythms**
   - Screen use, especially at night, suppresses melatonin, the sleep hormone, delaying sleep onset.
   - Poor sleep impairs function of the mood and memory centre, the hippocampus, affecting memory and learning.
   - Chronic sleep loss is also linked to reduced brain volume, ie fewer nerve cells in areas involved in emotional regulation.

6. **Effects on the Developing Brain Are Stronger in Younger Children**
   - In early childhood, screen exposure is linked with:
     - ○ Language delays.
     - ○ Weaker social skills.
     - ○ Reduced grey matter, ie nerve cells in key language and motor areas in the brain leading to delayed language and impaired mobility.

Neurochemical or Brain Chemical Messenger abnormalities

1. **The Reward Hijack: Dopamine Overload**
   - Dopamine is the brain's "feel-good" neurotransmitter.
   - Every like, comment, or notification releases a small dopamine burst, especially in the brain's reward centre.
   - Repeated stimulation causes:

- Desensitisation – the brain needs more screen time for the same pleasure.
- Reduced motivation for everyday tasks (eg homework, chores).
- Increased cravings, similar to addiction pathways.

2. **Cortisol: Increased Stress Response**
   - Constant online stimulation, fear of missing out (FOMO), and online conflict can raise cortisol, the stress hormone.
   - Chronic cortisol elevation can:
     - Impair memory and attention (especially in the Mood and Memory Centre, the hippocampus).
     - Affect sleep and emotional regulation.
     - Increase anxiety, especially in teens.

3. **Melatonin Suppression: Sleep Hormone Disrupted**
   - Blue light from screens (especially at night) suppresses melatonin, the hormone that helps children fall asleep.
   - Poor sleep leads to:
     - Reduced concentration and learning.
     - Lower emotional resilience.
     - Disruption of the brain's day night rhythm.

4. **Reduced Serotonin: Mood and Emotional Regulation**
   - Serotonin helps regulate mood, appetite, and sleep.
   - Screen overuse and lack of outdoor activity can lower serotonin levels due to:
     - Less natural light exposure.
     - Poor sleep.
     - Decreased physical activity.

- This can lead to:
  - Mood swings.
  - Irritability.
  - Sadness or low motivation.

5. **Imbalanced GABA and Glutamate: Focus and Calm**
   - GABA (calming neurotransmitter) and glutamate (stimulating neurotransmitter) need to stay balanced.
   - Overstimulation from fast-paced games or apps can lead to:
     - Excess glutamate, making children hyper-aroused and restless.
     - Reduced GABA, lowering the brain's ability to calm down and focus.

I hope you will agree with me that the snapshot of evidence that I have listed clearly demonstrates that excessive Smartphone, Device and Social media use, ie too much screen time, is associated with very worrying effects on the brain.

The Screen Demic has caused great harm to a whole generation of children and teenagers, but thanks to neuroplasticity there is definite and tangible hope for repair and recovery spearheaded by regular physical activity.

In the next chapter I am going to explore how physical activity can reverse many of these changes.

CHAPTER 12

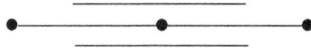

How Physical activity can reverse the brain changes due to excessive screens and social media use in children and teenagers

In the last 15 years, the Screen Demic has completely upended civilisation as we know it, not because of technology per se, but because far too many people have become addicted to smartphones, devices and social media apps.

Many of these people have unhealthy changes in the brain due to excessive screen time and social media use.

However, the good news is that neuroscience shows us that regular physical activity can reverse or offset many of these physical and neurochemical changes by boosting brain growth, connectivity, and function.

Let's look at some of the benefits with the evidence

Physical changes due to Physical activity

1. Focus, Planning, Self-Control centre (Rebuilding the Prefrontal Cortex)

- Exercise increases the size of the prefrontal cortex by increasing the number of nerve cells which helps improve:
  ○ Attention span.
  ○ Impulse control.

This region is underdeveloped in children with excessive screen exposure but strengthened through aerobic activity like running, biking, football cricket, rugby etc.

- *Evidence:* A nine-month exercise study showed greater prefrontal thickness, ie more nerve cells and improved cognitive control in children aged 7–9 (Hillman et al, 2014).

2. Repairing White Matter Connectivity

- White matter tracts are like highways connecting different brain areas.
- Excessive screen use disrupts myelination (the insulation) around nerves and leads to less organised white matter.
- Physical activity enhances white matter insulation and strength – especially in areas involved in:
  ○ Reading.
  ○ Language.

Evidence: Children who exercised regularly showed improved white matter structure in brain's connecting pathways (Chaddock-Heyman et al 2018).

3. Normalising the Reward System (The Striatum)

- The striatum, part of the emotional control circuitry, becomes hyperactive with screen use, reinforcing addictive behaviours.

- Physical activity helps rebalance and decrease reward hypersensitivity.
- This reduces screen cravings and enhances motivation for real-world activities.

Evidence: Studies show that exercise restores striatal function and improves motivation and self-regulation in teens (Belcher et al 2020).

4. **Increase in the number of nerve cells of the Emotional Control and Empathy centre (Anterior Cingulate Cortex)**
   - Exercise increases thickness by increasing the number of nerve cells in areas responsible for empathy, and emotional regulation.

Evidence: Children who engaged in regular physical education had increased grey matter, ie more nerve cells in the anterior cingulate, improving emotional intelligence (Ruotsalainen et al 2019).

5. **Restoring the size of the Mood and Memory Centre (The Hippocampus)**
   - Screens especially at night reduce hippocampal function by disrupting sleep.
   - Exercise increases nerve growth hormones such as BDNF (brain-derived neurotrophic factor) and IGF-1, hormones that lead to neurogenesis or the formation of more neurons in the hippocampus.

This improves memory, learning, and emotional regulation.

Evidence: Aerobic activity increases hippocampal volume and improves memory performance in children and adolescents (Chaddock et al 2010).

Physical activity acts like a neurochemical reset button — helping the brain recover from the damage caused by digital overstimulation.

1. **Rebalancing Dopamine: The Motivation Molecule**
   - Problem with screens: Social media and gaming flood the brain with dopamine, causing cravings and dependence.
   - How exercise helps: Physical activity provides a healthy dopamine boost without overstimulation.

Evidence: Regular aerobic activity increases dopamine levels and enhances mood, motivation, and attention, especially in children with attention difficulties (Meeusen & De Meirleir 1995).

2. **Boosting Serotonin: The Mood Stabiliser**
   - Problem with screens: Screen overuse and isolation reduce natural serotonin release, leading to irritability, sadness, or depression.
   - How exercise helps: Physical activity – especially outdoors – increases serotonin production and improves emotional balance.

Evidence: Moderate-to-intense exercise elevates serotonin levels, acting as a natural antidepressant (Chaouloff et al 1989).

3. **Restoring Melatonin: The Sleep Hormone**
   - Problem with screens: Blue light from screens suppresses melatonin which is the hormone responsible for inducing sleep, making it harder to sleep.
   - How exercise helps: Physical activity regulates the body clock, increases natural melatonin production, and improves sleep quality.

Evidence: Physical activity improves sleep onset and duration by supporting healthy melatonin cycles (Kredlow et al 2015).

4. **Lowering Cortisol: The Stress Hormone**
    *   Problem with screens: constant alerts, multitasking, and online discord raise cortisol, which can damage the brain over time.
    *   How exercise helps: Movement, especially rhythmic aerobic activity (like swimming, football, jogging or cycling), reduces cortisol and boosts resilience to stress.

Evidence: Children who exercise regularly show lower baseline cortisol and recover faster from stress (Martikainen et al 2013).

5. **Raising GABA: The Brain calming neurochemical**
    *   Problem with screens: Overstimulation reduces GABA activity → more anxiety, impulsivity, and poor emotional control.
    *   How exercise helps: Especially mind-body activities like yoga or aerobic movement increase GABA levels in the brain.

Evidence: A single session of yoga or aerobic exercise can significantly increase GABA in the thalamus, improving mood and calmness (Streeter et al 2010).

6. **Increasing BDNF: The Brain's Growth Fertiliser**
    *   Problem with screens: Less physical stimulation reduces BDNF, a hormone that supports new brain cell growth.
    *   How exercise helps: Physical activity – especially moderate to vigorous – dramatically raises BDNF, promoting brain repair and neuroplasticity.

So as you can see, physical activity has a variety of well documented and researched beneficial effects on the brains of children and teenagers suffering the effects of the Screen Demic.

Physical activity offers an accessible and affordable solution to the serious and damaging effects of excessive screens whilst setting the child or teenager up for better long-term physical and mental health.

CHAPTER 13

Changes in the Brain Associated with Gaming Disorder

The debate about excessive screen time has focussed mainly on the Screen Demic related to excessive smartphone use, excessive device use and addiction to social media.

Gaming seems to have managed to escape the appropriate scrutiny and I am hoping to redress that by highlighting many of the issues associated with excessive gaming now medically known as Internet Gaming Disorder (IGD), with evidence attached.

Internet Gaming Disorder (IGD) is a recognized condition characterised by compulsive or uncontrolled use of online or video games, resulting in significant impairment in daily life – including school, sleep, relationships, and mental health.

Internet Gaming Disorder was officially recognized by the World Health Organization (WHO) in 2019.

Some of the common symptoms of Internet Gaming Disorder are as follows:

1. Preoccupation with gaming.
2. Withdrawal symptoms when not playing (irritability, anxiety, sadness).
3. Tolerance – needing to play more over time.
4. Loss of interest in other activities.
5. Continued use despite problems.

6. Deceiving others about how much they play.
7. Jeopardising opportunities (school, friendships, family life).

Who's Most at Risk?

Risk Factor	Explanation
Age 10–18	Teens are more susceptible due to brain development
Males > Females	Boys are more likely to game excessively
Lack of offline friendships	Social isolation increases dependence on gaming
ADHD, depression, or anxiety	Comorbid conditions heighten the risk
Lack of parental supervision	Less family structure increases screen time
Games with social or reward loops	Multiplayer, reward-heavy games are more addictive

Effects on Children and Teenagers

Area Affected	Impact
School	Drop in grades, missed homework, reduced focus
Sleep	Insomnia, delayed sleep, fatigue

Mood	Increased anxiety, depression, irritability
Relationships	Family conflict, withdrawal from friends
Physical health	Sedentary lifestyle, weight gain, headaches
Cognitive skills	Poor impulse control, executive dysfunction

Physical Changes in the Brains of Children and Teenagers Who Spend Long Hours Gaming

1. **Structural Brain Changes**

    The brain's reward centres (the Striatum and Nucleus Accumbens) which are located near the front of the brain are responsible for feelings of pleasure and motivation. These structures are heavily involved in processing both natural rewards like food and also in the reinforcing effects of addictive substances.

    *   Studies using sensitive and accurate MRI scans have shown that frequent gaming is associated with increased size of the nucleus accumbens, areas involved in:
        *   Reward processing.
        *   Motivation.
        *   Habit formation.
    *   Importantly, similar brain changes are seen in other addictive behaviours, meaning that compulsive gaming causes similar changes in the brain to those seen in other addictions.

Evidence: Kühn et al, 2011 Frequent adolescent gamers showed increased volume in the striatum, which correlated with the amount of time spent gaming.

2. **Changes in Brain Centre responsible for decision making and Impulse control (the Prefrontal Cortex)**
Reduced Grey Matter, ie reduced nerve cells in Prefrontal Cortex in Excessive Gamers.
Evidence: Yuan et al, 2011 – Adolescents with Internet Gaming Disorder (IGD) had reduced grey matter density, ie reduced nerve cells in the prefrontal cortex which was associated with poorer emotional regulation.

3. **Impaired Connectivity Between Brain Regions**
   - Long hours of gaming can affect the functional connectivity between brain regions.
   - In excessive gamers, studies have found:
     ◦ Weaker connections between the areas responsible for emotional control.

Evidence: Studies using MRI scans show reduced grey matter, ie a reduction in nerve cells in areas involved in emotional regulation, attention, and impulse control in young people with IGD (Lee et al 2018).

4. **Abnormalities of the Brain Centre responsible for Self-monitoring and conflict resolution (Anterior Cingulate Cortex ACC).**

Studies have shown reduced volume, ie fewer nerve cells and reduced activity in the ACC, which may relate to difficulty in regulating gaming behaviour or recognizing negative consequences.
Evidence: Zhou et al, 2011 – Adolescents with IGD showed abnormal structure in the ACC and insula, areas tied to self-awareness and impulse control.

Neurochemical changes in the brain associated with gaming disorder

Internet Gaming Disorder (IGD) is associated with distinct neurochemical and hormonal changes in the brain, particularly involving systems that regulate reward, motivation, stress, impulse control, and mood.

These changes mirror patterns seen in substance addiction, and help explain why gaming can become compulsive and difficult to regulate.

Neurochemical and Hormonal Changes in IGD

1. **Dopamine – Overactivation of the Reward System**
   - Repeated gaming leads to dopamine surges, reinforcing the behaviour (similar to substance addiction).
   - Over time, this may cause:
     - Reduced pleasure from natural rewards (eg social interaction, academic achievement).

Evidence: Kim et al, 2011 Modern brain scans (MRI and PET scans) in adolescents with IGD showed changes in some of the emotional control centres in the brain, similar to responses seen in drug addiction.

2. **Low Serotonin levels leading to Impaired Mood and Impulse Regulation**
   - Effect:
     - Lower levels of serotonin are observed in people with IGD, contributing to:
       - Poor impulse control.
       - Mood swings.
     - Increased vulnerability to depression and anxiety.

Evidence: Kim et al, 2011: Adolescents with IGD showed lower levels of a by-product of serotonin in the fluid surrounding the brain suggesting reduced serotonin production.

3. **Cortisol – Elevated Stress Hormone Levels due to an overactive Stress Response Centre: HPA Axis (Hypothalamic–Pituitary–Adrenal Axis)**
    - Effect:
        ◦ Excessive gaming and sleep deprivation stimulate the HPA axis, increasing cortisol levels.
        ◦ Chronic elevation may impair:
            ▪ Sleep quality.
            ▪ Immune function.
            ▪ Emotional stability.

Evidence: Geisel et al 2015 showed high cortisol or stress hormone levels in adolescents with Internet Gaming Disorder.

4. **Norepinephrine – The fight and flight hormone**
    - Effect:
        ◦ Repetitive gaming, especially action or violent games, depletes norepinephrine levels.
    - This matters because norepinephrine helps regulate alertness, stress response, attention, and emotional control.
    - *Evidence:* Kim et al 2016 showed reduced norepinephrine levels in gamers.

5. **Oxytocin: Social Bonding Hormone released during acts of affection**
    - Effect:

- ○ Individuals with IGD may show blunted oxytocin responses during social interactions.
- ○ This impairs:
  - Empathy.
  - Social connectedness.
  - Interest in real-life relationships.

So as you can see there is now clear and abundant evidence proving conclusively that excessive gaming – which is meant by more than two hours per day of gaming consistently – can be associated with a wide range of abnormal physical and chemical changes in the brain.

Worryingly, the evidence tells us that these changes are similar to those individuals with other addictions, and even though Internet Gaming Disorder has gone under the radar of public awareness, all is not lost.

Please turn to the next chapter to understand how physical activity can reverse these physical, chemical and hormonal changes.

CHAPTER 14

Physical activity as treatment for Internet Gaming Disorder

Regular physical activity activates the brain's ability to rewire and heal itself. In children and teenagers with Internet Gaming Disorder (IGD), this leads to measurable structural and chemical improvements.

Physical Brain Changes from Physical Activity in Internet Gaming Disorder

1. Increased nerve cells (grey matter) in the Centre responsible for Emotional Regulation and Impulse control (Prefrontal Cortex)
   - What it means: Improved control over impulses, better decision-making, and stronger resistance to cravings.
   - *Evidence: Zhou et al 2021* found that aerobic exercise such as football, swimming, running and cycling etc increased prefrontal cortex volume, ie more nerve cells in adolescents with IGD.

2. Improved Communication pathways in the brain (White Matter Integrity)
   - What it means: Better communication between brain regions, leads to improved emotional regulation

- *Evidence: Dong et al 2020* used state of the art brain scans and images and found enhanced white matter tracts in teenagers with IGD after 12 weeks of physical activity, especially in pathways, which are essential for behaviour regulation.

3. **Reduced size of Overactive Reward Regions (eg Nucleus Accumbens)**
   - What it means: Less compulsive gaming, improved balance in brain reward systems.
   - *Evidence: Liu et al 2020* showed a normalisation of hyperactive reward circuits in adolescents with IGD following regular aerobic exercises such as swimming, running or cycling and team sports etc. This helps reduce the over-sensitivity to gaming stimuli and helps tackle the gaming addiction.

4. **Increased volume in the Memory and Mood Centre (The Hippocampus)**
   - What it means: More nerve cells leads to better memory, learning, and emotional processing.
   - *Evidence:* Studies in both healthy and IGD-affected youth (*Kuhn et al 2014; Park et al 2022*) demonstrate that physical activity increases hippocampal size.

Key Neurochemical and Hormonal Improvements from Physical Activity in IGD

1. **Dopamine – Rebalanced Reward System**
   - IGD Problem: Gaming overstimulates dopamine release, creating an addictive feedback loop.

- Exercise Effect: Moderate aerobic exercise boosts natural dopamine production, but in a controlled, sustainable way.
- Result: Reduces cravings for gaming and improves motivation for real-life activities.
- *Evidence: Wang et al 2019* found improved and reset dopamine levels after 12 weeks of aerobic training in adolescents with IGD.

2. **Serotonin – Improved Mood and Sleep**
   - IGD Problem: Sedentary behaviour and excessive gaming lower serotonin, increasing risk of depression.
   - Exercise Effect: Improved mood, emotional regulation, and sleep.
   - *Evidence:* Studies (*Kim et al 2020*) show exercise elevates serotonin levels and reduces depressive symptoms in youth with IGD.

3. **Cortisol – Reduced Stress**
   - IGD Problem: Chronic gaming and poor sleep elevate cortisol, the stress hormone.
   - Exercise Effect: Regular physical activity helps reduce cortisol levels over time.
   - Result: Lower anxiety, improved focus, and better regulation of emotions.
   - *Evidence: Liu et al 2018* reported decreased salivary cortisol (which is a reliable measure of this stress hormone) in adolescents with IGD after a structured exercise programme.

4. **Endorphins – Natural Pleasure Boosters**
   - IGD Problem: Endorphin release becomes dependent on gaming stimuli.

- Exercise Effect: Aerobic and moderate-intensity activity increases endorphins, leading to natural feelings of pleasure and reward.
- *Evidence:* Endorphin levels measured after exercise rise significantly in teens (*Hoffmann et al 2019*).

5. **Oxytocin – Enhanced Social Connection**
   - IGD Problem: IGD often results in social withdrawal and lower oxytocin (the bonding hormone).
   - Exercise Effect: Group sports and physical play boost oxytocin, enhancing trust and emotional connection.
   - Result: Rebuilds social relationships and improves emotional warmth.
   - *Evidence: Lee et al 2020* showed increased oxytocin levels in adolescents engaged in team-based exercise interventions.

6. **BDNF (Brain-Derived Neurotrophic Factor) – Brain Growth and Learning**
   - IGD is associated with: low levels of the nerve growth hormone BDNF leading to poorer learning, memory, and adaptability.
   - Exercise Effect: Physical activity increases BDNF, which supports the growth of new nerve cells and junctions between nerve cells.
   - Result: Enhanced learning capacity, emotional resilience, and brain recovery.
   - *Evidence: Huang et al 2021* found significantly elevated BDNF levels in IGD-affected youth after ten weeks of physical training.

Regular physical activity can lead to:
- Less craving and better control over gaming urges.
- Improved academic performance and focus.
- More emotional resilience and reduced anxiety.
- Healthier sleep and mood.
- Reconnection with family, peers, and real-life interests.

What Type of Exercise Works?

- Moderate to vigorous aerobic activity (eg running, swimming, football or any team sport): 45–60 minutes, 3–5 times/week.
- Activities that engage thinking and coordination (eg martial arts, team sports).
- Enjoyable routines your teenager will stick with (eg dance, cycling with friends).

Consistency over several weeks is key – most brain changes are noticeable after 8–12 weeks of regular physical activity.

Management and Treatment

At Home:
- Set daily screen time limits (ideally ≤ 1–2 hours/day).
- Establish screen-free zones (eg bedrooms, meals).
- Encourage physical activity, outdoor play, and family time.
- Use parental controls and supervise game content, however hard that might be.
- Model healthy digital habits.

Tips for Prevention

- Introduce children to balanced screen habits early (please remember parents are in charge of their children).
- Prioritise offline hobbies (music, sports, volunteering).
- Keep communication open and non-judgmental; however, be firm as and when needed.

Final Thoughts for Parents

- Exercise doesn't just have physical benefits, it is medicine for the brain.
- For teenagers struggling with Internet Gaming Disorder, physical activity can reverse harmful brain changes and restore mental health.

CHAPTER 15

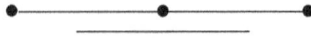

Tips for Tackling the Screen Demic

There is incontrovertible evidence that we are now submerged in a Screen Demic which I have defined earlier.

An unsuspecting population around the world have been hoodwinked into thinking that uncontrolled, unlimited and unfettered access to an opaque and often malevolent virtual world is benign and a force for good.

The reality is exactly the opposite, and in fact talking about unlimited and unfettered, let me introduce you to the version of TikTok available to Chinese people.

TikTok is owned by a Chinese company called Byte Dance. They offer a completely different version of TikTok in China, presumably because they are aware of the awful toxic effects associated with its use.

The Chinese version of TikTok is called Douyin and it is governed by the following rules:

- The App is not available between 10pm and 6am, ie no teenagers waking up to check the App due to FOMO.
- The content must be scientific, cultural with wholesome human stories, compared to the often misleading and poisonous content on TikTok
- Moderators ensure that the content is appropriate and sanitised, whereas in the rest of the world it is the Wild West.
- Influencers are BANNED!! Hallelujah.

Need I say more!

The world over parents and families have been misled into thinking that giving infants and young children devices and screens is actually good for them.

There is nothing further from the truth. Watching a screen is a passive process, hypnotising yes but completely passive, with the child condemned to watching a screen that provides flashing images and sounds.

A child cannot learn language and interaction from a screen – all of that **has** to come from family and friends and there is a huge amount of evidence conclusively proving the detrimental effects on early childhood due to excessive time spent on screens.

So what do I recommend in early childhood?

The book does contain a Five a Day Infographic which is a guide for parents, children and families about sensible and reasonable Screen Use; however, I will mention a couple for early childhood here.

Between the ages of 0-2 years, the only screen time should be video chatting.

Between the ages of 2 and 5 years the maximum daily screen time should be 30 minutes, preferably of educational content

Now of course bringing up children is not easy and there are times when parents will be forced to use a smartphone or device to keep a child quiet.

However, a smartphone or a device is NOT a Digital Dummy or a Digital Babysitter, and giving an infant or young child a smartphone more than the recommended time can be associated with a number of problems such as:

Poor language skills including the advent of non-verbal children, inability to regulate emotions, ie temper tantrums, impaired ability to interact with others, issues with mobility and posture as well as increased frequency of young children requiring glasses.

What about Teenagers?

A statistic to set the scene first: Teenagers seem to be spending less time with friends and Ofcom says the average British 11 or 12-year-old now spends 29 hours a week online, equivalent to almost a full-time job!

I am sure you will agree with me that cannot be healthy.

Neuroscience research has revealed that adolescence is a window of opportunity for learning and growth. Interactions, including school, family and peers (both online and offline), play a significant role in shaping the developing adolescent brain.

Adolescence is a period of life in which our sense of self, and particularly our sense of social self – that is, how others see us – undergoes a profound transition. As teenagers become more conscious of how others perceive them, they often experience increased self-consciousness and self-criticism.

Friends and peers have a huge influence too. Teenagers are especially sensitive to social rejection, so a lot of their choices revolve around fitting in and avoiding being excluded. This is what is called avoiding social risk – that is, the risk of being left out.

Social media can amplify this. With every post, like and comment, young people have to navigate a cycle of self-presentation and comparison, shaping their identities based on the curated, filtered lives fed to them by social media algorithms. Young people's evolving sense of self and what society expects of them are influenced and distorted by what they are exposed to both offline and online.

So the question is why do we allow our teenagers unfettered access to the wild west of the virtual world? We don't let 14-year-olds sign up for credit cards because we recognize that children are still developing their ability to make long-term decisions, yet we allow them to independently enter into contracts with large corporations – signing away the rights to their habits, thoughts and images – without ensuring they understand the implications.

This lack of protection is striking, with ten-year-olds routinely lying in order to access platforms, and many younger teenagers often receiving unwanted sexual content.

Here are some suggestions for children and adolescents aimed at Tackling the Screen Demic that has virtually infected our lives.

Not giving your child a smartphone is the new "my kids don't have sugar" for children.

Swap your child's smartphone for a dumbphone or a retro phone without the social media apps but for those parents who want to know where their children are all the time with GPS tracking capability.

Turn off notifications and make your phone monochrome or introduce greyscale into your phone.

If you have already given your child a smartphone, consider the following app blockers that actually work, Brick (£45) or Padlock (£34.49). These are palm-sized devices that you tap against your iPhone to temporarily remove distracting apps and then stash somewhere out of the way.

You can then reinstall them as a reward on occasion.

For children who have a smartphone, ensure regular non-tech breaks – it could be looking at a wall, staring out of the window, stretching, going for a walk, involving the children in housework, taking the dog for a walk, walking to and from school – the key is not to be productive or feed the brain with any more information.

Parents should make a deal with their children when they are given their first mobile phone that it will not be kept by their bedside.

Smart kids don't take Smartphones to bed!

Supporting Your Child

Have meaningful conversations at the dinner table or in the car

Being heard and valued in family conversations boosts a child's confidence and sense of responsibility. It reassures them that their opinions matter, empowering them to express themselves more freely not just at home, but in school and social settings as well.

Give them ownership over everyday decisions

We tend to take away ownership and control from children. Giving a child a choice of which pair of socks they're going to put on, what they're going to do that day or what they will eat for tea that night is giving them power over their life and confidence in their ability to navigate it.

Brainstorm rather than offer solutions to scary situations

Children can prefer the virtual world to the real one because it can feel less scary. Have conversations with your children about the things that scare them. Instead of providing solutions, encourage them to share their ideas and help them put those into practice.

"Is there anything you would like to change about your family?" or "What chores would you like to do?". These conversations allow children to consider different perspectives, express their thoughts and navigate emotions with the support of loved ones.

Talk to your child, especially teenagers, about the decisions they face and the options they are considering. Help them to identify any blind spots in their choices without stating your preference or coercing them. Be non-judgmental, but use your wisdom if something feels wrong or dangerous.

Show them – don't tell them – how to make difficult decisions

Decision-making is not hardwired but involves skills that can be learnt, such as other critical thinking skills. Model good decision behaviour, such as evaluating pros and cons and avoiding decisions in highly emotional states. Focus on how decisions are made rather than the outcomes.

Give your children household tasks

Children like to feel that they are givers, not just takers, and one way to give at home is to share the domestic jobs.

Provide regular routines. Children with dependable schedules which included set family mealtimes, regular playtimes with their parents and bedtime stories in the evening were also more likely to get more sleep than those with less structure in their lives.

What about outside the house?

A survey by OnePoll in 2022, for the charity Play England, found that 27 per cent of children regularly play outside their homes, compared with 80 per cent of adults aged between 55 and 64 today, when they were children. Parents cited stranger danger and traffic as their main reasons for stopping their children playing outdoors.

Collaborate with neighbours to 'kick the kids outdoors'

Arrange a certain time every weekend or one day a week after school with neighbours to act like old-fashioned parents and encourage your children out of the house – and keep their phones inside.

Most children are innately drawn to other kids to play with. If there is concern about safety, the group could have an adult chaperone, just to watch for emergencies, not to intervene in the play.

Let them have sleepovers and don't micromanage

Sleepovers have become less popular with some families over the years amid fears that their children could be hurt, scared or exposed to things they shouldn't see. In doing so, we are underestimating them and overestimating danger. Sleepovers are great for bonding and getting used to being away from your parents. It's also so interesting for kids to see how another family lives, has fun and makes breakfast etc.

Don't drive your children everywhere

Independent mobility is a great confidence builder. Think about errands your child might do for you.

Go on outdoor adventures – and hand over the reins When you go on adventures such as camping, give the children tasks they can complete without adults, such as putting up a small tent. It takes away that sense of being wrapped in cotton wool and instils confidence.

MORE GREEN TIME LESS SCREEN TIME is the Mantra!

Encourage teenagers to get a paying job outside the home

This helps teenagers to feel more grown up and confident about their future. They learn that they can be responsible and earn their own money, so adulthood seems less scary. Their own money is itself a further ticket to independence.

I hope you will agree with me that in most families many of these suggestions are not difficult to implement

Whatever approach you adopt for your family, particularly when dealing with the poisonous and addictive effects of the Screen Demic, remember that whilst it is not going to be easy implementing change and enforcing moderation, in the end it will all be worth it because control over the phone rather than vice versa will go a long way towards securing your child's future.

One final thought that will hopefully help you in the battle for moderation and escaping the phone-based and phone-controlled childhood is that as the parent ultimately you are in charge and the short term pain will most definitely lead to long term gain for your child and your family!

CHAPTER 16

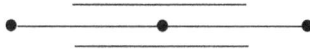

Why Sunlight Matters for children and teenagers with Mental Health Disorders

Sunlight is the most potent trigger for the production of Vitamin D; it is certainly more effective than taking oral supplements.

Vitamin D in turn has a number of important roles in brain function, some of which I have listed below:

1. **Helps Build and Protect Brain Cells**
   Vitamin D activates genes that grow new nerve cells and protects existing ones.

2. **Supports Key Brain Chemicals**
   Vitamin D regulates the production of dopamine and serotonin – neurochemicals involved in mood, motivation, and focus.

3. **Reduces Inflammation in the Brain**
   Chronic inflammation can damage brain tissue over time.

   Vitamin D has anti-inflammatory effects, calming the brain's immune cells and protecting against damage.

4. **Boosts Brain Energy**
   Vitamin D influences how brain cells use glucose (the brain's main fuel) and supports the brain's energy batteries (mitochondria).

What are Skin-Brain Pathways?

When sunlight hits the skin, it triggers multiple responses:
- Vitamin D production → supports brain development, mood, and cognition.
- β-Endorphin release → natural "feel-good" chemicals that boost mood (similar to the runner's high).

Sunlight isn't a cure – but growing evidence shows that it is a powerful boost for brain development, mood, attention, and sleep in children with ADHD, Autism and other mental health disorders in children and adolescents. When paired with physical activity and healthy routines, it forms part of a broader strategy to support their well-being.

The Effect of Sunlight on Mental Health Conditions

1. **Sunlight Supports Mood through Natural Light Exposure**
   - Sunlight helps the brain make serotonin – the "feel-good" neurotransmitter that boosts mood and focus.
   - Research shows that serotonin levels are higher on sunny days than on cloudy ones, regardless of the temperature.

Evidence: Lambert et al (2002): found that serotonin levels in the brain was directly related to the amount of sunlight exposure – more sunlight = more serotonin.

2. **Outdoor Light and Time in Nature Improves Emotional Well-being**
   Overviews of research evidence indicate that time spent in natural settings – parks, gardens, forests, consistently leads to lower stress, reduced depressive symptoms, and improved resilience in children and teens (Shanahan et al 2016).

3. **Sunlight Resets Circadian Rhythms and Sleep**
   - Bright sunlight exposure – especially in the morning – helps stabilise the body's sleep-wake (circadian) rhythms.
   - Since disrupted sleep is common in ADHD, better sleep can reduce irritability, impulsivity, and inattention (Figueiro et al 2013).

Final Takeaway

Sunlight and natural light don't replace therapy, but research tells us that adequate daylight exposure, especially in the morning along with time outdoors, plays a meaningful role in supporting healthy mood, sleep, and emotional well-being in teens.

I do wonder since humanity exists because of the sun and sunlight, why don't we make more use of such a ready-made therapy for mental health disorders.

Why Winter Can Be Hard for Children's Mental Health
- Shorter days and less sunlight can lower serotonin levels (the "feel-good" brain chemical).
- Cold weather often means less outdoor play, leading to more screen time, isolation, and mood dips.

- Some kids develop Seasonal Affective Disorder (SAD) – a form of depression linked to reduced daylight.

How Winter Activities Help

1. **Boosts Mood Chemicals**
   - Physical activity – even in winter – triggers the release of endorphins, dopamine, and serotonin.
   - These brain chemicals act like natural antidepressants, helping lift mood and ease anxiety.

2. **Regulates Stress and Sleep**
   - Exercise lowers cortisol, the stress hormone.
   - It also helps reset the body clock, improving sleep, crucial for children with anxiety or depression.

3. **Keeps Children Socially Connected**
   - Winter activities (eg ice skating, indoor sports, group games, team sports) offer social contact, which protects against isolation – a major factor in depression.

4. **Counters "Winter Slump"**
   - Movement, even indoors, fights the sluggishness that shorter days bring.
   - Children who stay active in winter report more energy, better focus, and less irritability.

How winter activities help children with ADHD and Autism

- Short bouts of aerobic activity (like running or dance) enhance cognition in children with ADHD by improving brain function, even in winter settings.

- Outdoor or indoor winter activities help release dopamine and norepinephrine, aiding attention and emotional regulation.
- For children with autism, sensory-rich outdoor or indoor play supports motor development, emotional regulation, and stress relief, even in cold months.
- An overview of numerous studies showed that structured exercise benefits – including social skills, behaviour, and executive function – hold for children with autism even during colder months, and I have covered the evidence in quite a lot of detail in the previous chapters.

Here are some ideas to stay active in the winter

Trampoline	Offers energy release and helps with balance – especially helpful for ADHD
Dance sessions	Engages the brain, coordinates movement, and lifts mood
Yoga or martial arts	Supports sensory processing, self-regulation, and emotional control
Sledging, snow play	Combines fun, movement, and social interaction when weather allows

My own structured year-round activity is karate and even though going to the dojo in the cold of winter can feel like a drag, once I've done the warming routine the sessions are always rewarding and invigorating.

Being active in winter is one of the strongest natural tools for helping kids manage the entire range of mental health disorders in childhood and adolescence.

As a well-known Swedish American psychologist said, 'there is no such thing as bad weather just bad clothes'.

CHAPTER 17

•———————•———————•

The Benefits of Physical Activity on Sleep

The brain is the most active and metabolically demanding organ in the human body. It consumes a significant amount of energy, roughly 20% of the body's total calorie intake, despite only making up about 2% of the body's weight. This high energy demand is essential for the brain's complex functions and constant activity.

Given the multitude and complexity of the brain's functions, nature has designed a mechanism by which it recuperates from all its activities.

That happens during sleep.

Sleep is one of the most important bodily functions and until recently probably one of the least understood.

We now know that sleep is a very active process during which the brain recovers from its significant workload during the day.

In addition, it is the time when toxic waste products produced during the preceding hours get excreted, memories get embedded, and the brain rests, regenerates and recuperates from the day's activities.

Crucially, it allows the brain to prepare for optimal performance the next day.

Good sleep and sleep of an adequate duration is essential for overall well-being, ie both brain health and physical health.

As a rough guide, a newborn should sleep 12-14 hours which reduces to 9-10 hours in early childhood and to 7-8 hours in teenagers and in adults.

Getting enough quality sleep is essential for children and teenagers as sleep plays a crucial role in brain development, physical growth, emotional regulation, learning, and behaviour. Unfortunately, many young people today are not getting the sleep they need – and the consequences can be significant.

The most common reason children are not getting enough sleep is excessive smartphone, device and social media use.

As if the brain doesn't have enough of a workload, subjecting the brain to hours of flashing images, reels etc is causing brain strain.

The brain is not a muscle, but just like a muscle it needs to rest and recover, which is what happens during sleep. In fact, during the day even a short nap can be restorative for the brain.

Poor sleep is associated with a multitude of problems in children and teenagers, such as difficulty concentrating, behavioural issues, mood swings, and impaired cognitive function.

Chronic sleep deprivation can also increase the risk of anxiety, depression, and even suicidal thoughts. In addition, sleep problems can negatively impact academic performance and increase the likelihood of risky behaviours.

Regular physical activity has a profoundly positive impact on sleep in children and adolescents. The relationship between movement and sleep is bidirectional: exercise helps improve sleep quality, and good sleep supports better physical performance, emotional regulation, and academic success.

1. Improved Sleep Duration

Studies consistently show that children and teens who engage in moderate to vigorous physical activity tend to sleep longer at night. Exercise increases the body's need for rest and recovery, helping regulate the body clock whilst promoting earlier sleep onset.

Evidence: A 2020 overview of available research evidence by Jansenn et al found that regular physical activity was associated with an increase of about 18 minutes of sleep per night in children and adolescents.

On the other hand,

- A study in 2014 by Magee et al concluded that every hour of sedentary behaviour was linked to reduced sleep duration, more evidence that excessive screen time is not good for children and adolescents, while increased physical activity correlated with longer sleep.

2. Faster Sleep Onset

Children who are more physically active tend to fall asleep more quickly. This is likely due to increased energy expenditure and a calming effect on the nervous system.

Evidence: Alnawwar et al in 2023 demonstrated that physically active adolescents reported significantly shorter time to fall asleep than their less active peers.

3. Better Sleep Quality

Physical activity enhances sleep efficiency (percentage of time in bed spent asleep), reduces night-time awakenings, and increases deep sleep, which is essential for brain development and memory consolidation.

Evidence:

- A 2021 study by Fonseca et al concluded that children who exercised regularly had less fragmented sleep and higher sleep efficiency.
- Aerobic activities like running, swimming, or cycling etc were particularly linked to better deep sleep in multiple studies.

4. Regulation of Circadian Rhythms

Exercise, particularly when done in the morning or early afternoon, helps optimise the body's internal clock (circadian rhythm), promoting consistent bed and wake times.

Evidence: Kredlow et al (2015): Reviewed 34 studies and found that acute and regular exercise improved several sleep metrics, particularly when not done close to bedtime.

- In addition, exposure to natural light during outdoor activity also supports the body clock, especially important for teens whose wake sleep cycles tend to change later in puberty.
- In other words, more green time less screen time is the way to go.

5. Reduced Sleep Disorders

Physical activity is linked to a lower risk of insomnia, sleep-disordered breathing, and other paediatric sleep disturbances.

Evidence: Bornsdottir et al 2024 reviewed the habits of 4399 adolescents and found physically active teenagers had a lower risk of insomnia symptoms and extreme sleep durations.

Davis et al 2006 showed that regular exercise helps in reducing symptoms of obstructive sleep apnoea (OSA) in overweight children.

6. Mental Health Benefits

Exercise reduces stress, anxiety, and symptoms of depression – all of which are linked to poor sleep. By enhancing mood and reducing cortisol (the stress hormone), physical activity prepares the body and mind for restful sleep.

Evidence: Alnawwar et al in 2022 did a systematic review of the available research which found that children who are physically active have lower levels of anxiety and depression, which in turn contributes to significantly better sleep outcomes.

7. Enhanced Daytime Functioning

With improved sleep comes better daytime alertness, concentration, behaviour, and emotional regulation – creating a positive cycle where good sleep enables better participation in physical activity and vice versa.

Evidence: Gruber et al (2012) – Children who had even one hour less sleep had significantly worse emotional regulation and behaviour in school.

Important Notes:
- Avoid vigorous exercise close to bedtime, as it may stimulate the nervous system and delay sleep.
- Regularity is key, benefits are best when activity is sustained over weeks or months.

Conclusion

Physical activity is a powerful, natural intervention that enhances sleep in children and young people. It improves sleep quality, duration, and onset, optimises the body clock and reduces the risk of sleep disorders.

These sleep benefits, in turn, support cognitive, emotional, and physical health – underscoring the importance of making exercise a daily habit in childhood and adolescence.

The concept of sleep hygiene is crucial to the health and well-being of children of any age.

I would strongly recommend NO screens in the Under Fives, two hours before bedtime; and for 6-17 year olds I would strongly advise no screens at least one hour before bedtime, with phones being put on silent and/or charged outside the bedroom during the night.

A good night's sleep is one of the most powerful tools for your child's growth and well-being. Put simply: children who sleep well are happier, healthier, and better able to thrive each day.

CHAPTER 18

—•———•———•—

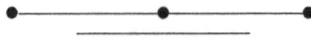

How Physical Activity Improves Gut Health in Children and Teenagers

I am sure you have heard a lot about gut health recently with good reason.

Previously the gut was a relatively unexplored and undiscovered organ; in fact, traditionally it was viewed mainly as the body's food waste pipe.

Recently, however, scientists are learning and unearthing so much more about this ecosystem within our bodies that I decided to spend some time exploring this topic.

Why Gut Health Matters

The gut is home to trillions of bacteria (the gut microbiome), some good, some potentially harmful, that play a critical role in:

- Digesting food.
- Regulating the immune system.
- Producing vitamins.
- Influencing brain health via the Brain Gut axis.

A healthy gut supports physical and mental health while an unhealthy one can contribute to problems such as poor immunity, anxiety, ADHD symptoms, mood disorders, and even obesity.

Let's take a quick look at how physical activity helps Gut Health and the Brain Gut axis.

What Is the Brain-Gut Axis?

The brain-gut axis is the two-way communication system between the brain and the digestive system (gut). It is made up of:

- Nerves (like the vagus nerve which links the brain to the gut).
- Hormones (like cortisol and serotonin).
- Chemical Signals.
- Gut bacteria.

This Axis helps regulate mood, thinking, digestion, immunity, and even sleep.

How Physical Activity Helps the Brain-Gut Axis

Regular physical activity helps this brain-gut connection work better by influencing several important components:

1. Activates the Vagus Nerve – The Main Gut-Brain Messenger

- What it does: The vagus nerve links the brain to the gut, an odd channel of communication you might think, but please do remember that the human body, being such an incredible creation, is still quite a mystery, and despite the breathtaking progress in technology we are still discovering how the human body works.

- Exercise effect: Moderate physical activity (like brisk walking or cycling) stimulates this nerve, improves digestion, and regulates emotions
- Result: Children feel calmer, have better gut function, and improved mood.
- *Evidence:* Christensen et al 2010 – Demonstrated that vagus nerve activity is enhanced after regular aerobic activity, improving both emotional regulation and digestion.

2. Improves Gut Microbiome and provides Healthy Brain Signals

- What happens: regular exercise increases the number and variety of "good" gut bacteria like Bifidobacteria and Lactobacillus. Probiotics have plenty of these healthy bacteria hence the recent surge in interest.
- Guess what: you can produce more healthy bacteria just through physical exercise!

So why is it important to have good bacteria in the gut?

Good bacteria

- Produce an acid called lactic acid which inhibits harmful bacteria.
- Enhance the intestinal barrier, preventing "leaky gut".
- Produce antibacterial substances that directly kill harmful germs.
- In addition, the good bacteria produce chemicals (called short-chain fatty acids) that send signals to the brain to increase the production of neurochemicals like serotonin.

- Physical activity increases the diversity and health of gut bacteria which in turn produce more of these chemicals that act on the brain.
- Why it matters: Healthy bacteria make the brain more resilient to stress, anxiety, and depression and in addition gut bacterial diversity improves digestion, reduces inflammation, and supports a stronger immune system.
- Result: children have better emotional control and fewer gut complaints.
- *Evidence: Estaki et al 2016* and *Clarke et al 2014* showed young adults who exercise regularly have more diverse and balanced gut bacteria than inactive peers.

3. Reduces Stress Hormones - Calms the Gut and Brain

- What it does: high levels of cortisol (the stress hormone) can disrupt both gut function as well as lowering the mood.
- Exercise effect: regular movement helps reduce cortisol and increase feel-good hormones like endorphins.
- Why it matters: this improves digestion, and supports emotional regulation.
- Result: children feel less anxious and have fewer stomach aches due to constipation.
- *Evidence:* Kochli et al 2021 showed physical activity significantly lowered cortisol levels.

4. Boosts Serotonin - The Mood and Gut Motility Messenger

- 95% of serotonin, the chemical responsible for so many brain functions and associated with so much malfunction when the levels are low, is made in the gut. Serotonin also has a role in gut function.

- Exercise effect: Physical Activity increases serotonin levels in both the brain and gut.
- Why it matters: helps with both mood and bowel movement regularity.
- Result: fewer mood swings and better digestion (Vazquez Medina et al 2024)

5. Reduces Inflammation in the Gut

- What happens: exercise lowers levels of chemicals in the gut that cause inflammation.
- Why it matters: this helps protect the structure of the gut and reduces the risk of gut-related issues like irritable bowel syndrome (IBS) and a leaky gut.
- *Evidence: Petersen & Pedersen 2005* showed that moderate exercise reduces inflammation in the entire body as well as the gut.

6. Improves Gut Motility (Movement)

- What happens: physical activity helps stimulate intestinal muscle contractions, promoting smoother and more regular bowel movements.
- Why it matters: it prevents constipation and encourages the healthy movement of food and waste
- *Evidence:* Matsuzaki *et al 2018* found that exercise significantly improved gut transit time in children with functional constipation.

Recommendations for Parents

- Encourage at least 30 minutes of moderate physical activity three to four days per week (eg cycling, swimming, playing outdoors etc).
- Support hydration, at least five to six glasses of a liquid (preferably water) a day and a fibre-rich diet alongside exercise.
- Activities like yoga, walking, or swimming are especially helpful for children with gut-related discomfort or anxiety.

In Summary

Encouraging physical activity in children and teenagers is a simple yet powerful way to promote a healthy gut, which can lead to numerous positive health outcomes throughout their lives, helping the brain as well as the body.

•————————•————————•

CHAPTER 19

An approach to Physical Activity: Suggestions for Parents

Physical activity is the best medicine for many reasons. It helps improve sleep, reduces stress, lifts the mood and concentration, and it can treat and prevent many medical problems pertaining to both mental and physical health. It also provides an opportunity for families to bond in healthy, memorable ways and if undertaken sensibly usually has no side effects, unlike medication!

Parents often think that in order to gain benefits from exercise, workouts must be intense or demanding. But research has shown that even short bouts of physical activity are beneficial.

The key is to try to make exercise fun for the whole family.

Here are a few suggestions for getting children outdoors and for adding more physical activity into daily life, and none of these involve spending vast sums of money.

1. Starting slowly

Going too hard too soon is the biggest problem people run into when starting to exercise. For most people, going from infrequent or little exercise to long periods of exercise is not going to be practical or sustainable. In addition, such an approach increases the risk of injuries.

Instead, start slowly, perhaps by taking short walks with your family. You can then increase the time and speed of the walks as you get comfortable. You can always add in more exercise as you go.

Another way to start slowly is to incorporate more movement into your daily activities: like taking the stairs rather than the lift. The more you encourage kids to move, the more likely you are to create a habit and help them be regularly active.

Taking the stairs is one of my favourite physical activities and as a routine I run up the stairs with my loaded briefcase to my office which, depending on which office it is, is either the 4th or 5th floor.

Now I didn't start by running up, I acclimatised myself by walking up and once comfortable began running up. I now never take the lift at work and elsewhere in life I minimise how much I use the lift. If I see an escalator I will try to run up it, be it at the tube station or the airport etc.

These short sharp bursts of activity are really good for both physical and mental health, and have certainly done wonders for my fitness.

Here are a few additional tips for incorporating physical activity into everyday routines, and the earlier you engage your children in these activities the more successful you are likely to be:

Homework
- Take five-minute breaks during homework time to move around, or get a standing desk so kids have the option to stand up during homework time.
- If the answer to the maths question is ten, your child could perhaps do ten jumping jacks; young children will potentially find this a lot of fun.
- Kitchen dance parties: put on some music and let them go full freestyle. (Bonus points if you join in!)

Obstacle courses at home, cushions, chairs, boxes – whatever you've got. It's amazing how exciting an indoor 'ninja course' can be on a rainy day.

Grocery shopping

- Park at the far end of the parking lot at the supermarket to get more steps in.
- Walk briskly, in fact speed walk to the supermarket and back whilst minding other cars and customers.
- Take extra trips through the aisles to move more while filling the trolley.

Going to school

- Walk or bike to school with your kids.
- Park a few streets away from school and walk them in or let them walk alone if they are old enough. Again, there is a huge amount of evidence about the benefits of brisk walking.
- You can even follow the Japanese walking technique of brisk walking for three minutes followed by relaxed walking for a few minutes then alternating the two.
- There are lots of proven health benefits of this too.

2. Define family exercise goals

Setting fitness goals is a great way to stay healthy together, but they don't have to be difficult. Start with a goal that you know you have time for and can achieve as a family.

For example, a family might decide to walk for 30 minutes a day, three days a week. Create a family calendar together so that as the ticked boxes accumulate, the family gains confidence and satisfaction in goals met.

Avoid making the physical activity too regimented and non-negotiable, ie don't put undue pressure on the kids to comply.

If they feel like missing the odd session that's fine, but then don't go and reward them with time on a smartphone device or gaming instead.

That must be a red line or it will keep tempting them into missing more and more family activity time together.

- Hold everyone accountable by setting a long-term family goal (such as running a 5K together).
- When you reach your family goal, consider a reward that encourages a commitment to physical activity, like getting new trainers.
- The key is to try to keep the activities going even in winter because there is no such thing as bad weather, just bad clothes for the weather.

3. Make family exercise enjoyable

One of the biggest obstacles people run into with fitness is thinking they have to do physical activities they don't enjoy. But exercise shouldn't feel like a chore. Some people like going running, but for those who don't, there are plenty of other ways to get in shape.

The best way to stick to an exercise regimen is finding something that you like, and the same goes for kids. The best physical activity for children is whatever they enjoy. Just get them active. It can be dancing, running, swimming, football, jumping rope, bike riding – anything that keeps them moving and helps build an active lifestyle.

The key to success is setting realistic goals, so avoid the usual New Year resolution fanatical fitness pledge of going to the gym five or six times per week for the rest of time, because that is not sustainable and will be demoralising when you are forced to give it up because it is too onerous!

Sound science tells us that regular physical activity three times a week has plenty of health benefits for the entire family.

Get kids active outdoors: More Green Time Less Screen Time

Research shows that spending time outdoors can reduce worry and promote a happier mood in children. In addition, the mental health benefits of exercise can provide positive physical outcomes, such as improved sleep and fewer anxiety-related stomach aches or headaches. As a result, children feel more energised and are then more willing to get outside and stay active.

Going Outdoors

Getting children active outdoors doesn't have to be a huge excursion – explore the options in your neighbourhood, such as walking, biking and hiking trails.

To make these outings even more fun, parents can add little games or challenges, such as spotting a certain animal or gathering leaves for a craft activity. Make a list of all the parks nearby and turn it into a summer mission to visit each one. Pack snacks, bring a ball, and let them run wild.

Make a list of exercise ideas

Another common misconception about exercise is that it requires paying for a gym membership or other expenses. But all you need to get kids active are activities that are exciting and accessible. Create a list of fun and free ways to stay fit and healthy. Allow your kids to choose from the list to help them get excited about the activity. For example, your list might look like the following:

- Let's go for a walk.
- It's time to get the bikes out and go for a ride.
- Let's go play football in the park near our house.

Explore free local activities. Libraries, museums, and councils often run summer programmes for little ones.

Water play in the garden. A bucket, a cup, a sponge. That's all you need. They'll pour, splash, run, and giggle their way to a nap-worthy level of tiredness.

- In addition around the country there are local Football Associations that offer training sessions for between £3 and £5 which, given how football mad we are as a country, should be accessible to most families.
- In fact, as Great Britain is always one of the most successful Olympic nations, having won over 60 medals in each of the last three games (with 32 sports in each games) there are a wide range of sporting activities available to everyone to participate in.

How to make time for exercise

Think about how you can incorporate regular physical activity into your daily life as a family. For example, consider the following activities:

- Kick a football around the garden or park for 30 minutes.
- Turn on some music and have a dance party.
- Take a 20-minute walk after dinner.
- Play a game of tag.
- Whether it's a local park or a walk around the block, set a challenge: can they spot a red door, a ladybird, a stick shaped like a Y.

Just spending time as a family and enjoying each other's company can take the focus off distractions and build bonds. It can also make doing activities as a family something parents and children look forward to.

4. Set a good example of family fitness

Children mirror the behaviour of the adults around them. Getting kids to eat fruit and vegetables, drink water instead of juice or soda, and increase their physical activity will be easier if parents lead by example.

Try modelling enthusiasm for health and exercise by sticking to the family-defined schedule and discussing the importance of exercise to your life and well-being. If you care deeply about physical fitness, chances are, your kids will, too.

5. Get plenty of sleep

Good sleep is vital for good health, and unlike what is commonly assumed, sleep is an active process during which the brain recovers and recharges from the day and for the next. Children who exercise sleep better as long as the exercise is not just before bedtime! Sleep can benefit other aspects of children's lives, too. Getting sufficient quality sleep is important for overall health, including school performance, behaviour and weight.

6. Limit screen time

Limiting screen time is important, but it can seem like a big challenge when so much of our day is filled with computers, televisions or tablets. I would recommend setting limits, rather than trying to eliminate screen time. When the time limit is up, you turn it off. Then you have more time to spend together as a family, and it can be fun.

Screen breaks are a great opportunity to get outside, and they can be done as a family to foster bonding. This can help everyone relax, make time for physical activity and feel more refreshed and focused to concentrate on school and work after the break. Additionally, you can schedule breaks to match screen time with outdoor time. For example, 30 minutes of screen time can equal 30 minutes of time outdoors.

Another fun idea is to incorporate physical activity challenges into screen time. For example, you can see how many jumping jacks, push-ups or sit-ups your family can do during a commercial break.

7. Maintaining a healthy weight range

Prioritising health and fitness goals as a family is also important for maintaining a healthy weight range. Remember: food is fuel. In the same way that a car needs the right fuel to run, healthy food fuels and energises our bodies to meet the demands of daily life. Eating well and maintaining a healthy weight range is also important for preventing illness and disease.

The earlier children start with building healthy habits, like eating a balanced diet and exercising, the easier it'll be to maintain these practices later in life.

Finally, please remember that parents are always in charge.

Whilst it might be easier to get your younger children to engage with a physical activity plan that you have set, it is probably going to be more difficult to get your teenagers to comply.

In that situation I would strongly urge you not to allow your teenager to substitute physical activity with a screen activity because you are allowing unhealthy habits to become entrenched.

Even if it means vetoing the screen activity for boredom, that's fine – boredom is much healthier for your teenager and there is now plenty of scientific evidence backing that up too!

CHAPTER 20

• ———— • ———— •

Back to the Future: How Physical Activity Leads to Long Term Resilience in Children and Adolescents

The importance of physical activity has been recognised for millennia – philosophers in Ancient Greece advocated the concept of "mens sana in corpore sano", a sound mind in a sound body, as the symbol of the balance between intellectual development, mental equilibrium, and physical activity, which constitute the core values of the human being.

Following that, during the Renaissance, there was a resurgence of interest in the connection between physical activity and mental health. In this period, the Italian physician and philosopher Mercuriale (1530–1606), in his book "The Art of Gymnastics Among the Ancients", published in 1569, laid the foundation for exercise principles based on the works of Greek and Roman authors. This book stressed that all healthy individuals should engage in regular physical exercise, forsake a sedentary lifestyle, and seek, through physical activity, the equilibrium between the body and the mind.

In 1800s England, Thomas Arnold introduced sports activities at Rugby School as a means of instilling values and to develop the character and personality of young students. Another enlightened thinker, Thomas Wood, argued in 1893 that physical education was a crucial means for the holistic development of children, significantly contributing to their emotional and intellectual growth. He published a book entitled 'Health by Stunts', perhaps the historical equivalent of today's parkour or rock climbing!

As you can see from the brief history above, knowledge of the connection between physical activity, sports, and psychological well-being has been present since the dawn of humanity; however, sadly and tragically, swathes of the population who have been entrapped by the addiction to smartphones devices and social media apps participate in very little physical activity.

As a result, the so-called Internet Revolution is contributing to the involution of the Human Mind and Body.

I am going to spend a little time exploring how physical activity and sports is intricately linked to long term resilience in children and teenagers.

Mental Resilience

Participating in team sports or group fitness activities fosters a sense of community and belonging, essential for emotional well-being. The support network provided by these communal activities plays a vital role in reducing feelings of isolation and loneliness, and participating in sports and physical activity leads to improved social skills and a stronger sense of community.

Achieving exercise goals, whether related to endurance, strength, or skills, leads to a sense of accomplishment and self-worth, which is particularly important for individuals with a low self-esteem and positively affects their overall mood and quality of life.

Physical activity cultivates psychological resilience by fostering skills such as teamwork, perseverance, and self-motivation; sports equip individuals with the tools necessary for effectively navigating life's adversities, thus contributing significantly to their long-term emotional and psychological well-being.

Discipline, a crucial ingredient of sports, educates individuals about dedication, persistence, and the management of failure, which are all essential for living in the real and very competitive world. The repetitive nature of training and commitment to improvement, despite setbacks, can translate into a more resilient approach to personal and professional challenges.

The multidimensional impact of physical activity and sports on emotional regulation is undeniable. Through the release of neurotransmitters and endorphins, exercise effectively enhances mood and mitigates stress, while fostering psychological resilience and well-being. The synthesis of physiological, psychological, and social benefits demonstrates the essential role of regular physical activity in maintaining and improving resilience.

Repeated mastery of physical challenges reinforces the belief: *"I can handle most situations in life."*

The literature shows that young people who regularly participate in sports activities also have significantly more physical resilience than those who do not participate.

Physical Resilience

Immune System Training

Moderate, regular exercise strengthens the immune system, lowering infection risk and speeding recovery.

Regular Physical Activity reduces chronic low-grade inflammation, which is linked to both physical illness and mood disorders.

Musculoskeletal Strength and Cardiovascular Health

Stronger muscles, bones, and heart mean the body can handle both physical stress (sports, injuries) and everyday demands with less fatigue.

Physical Activity leads to higher peak bone mass in adolescence, which protects against osteoporosis decades later and it also improves posture and balance, reducing injury risk.

Metabolic Resilience

Sustained improvements in insulin metabolism and lipid profiles protect against obesity, type 2 diabetes, and cardiovascular disease. Surely that is enough of an incentive to educate children about the benefits of physical activity from early childhood?

Sleep Quality

Regular physical activity improves sleep onset, depth, and regularity – critical for recovery and growth.

Healthy Coping Skills

Physically active children often develop positive outlets for stress (movement, play) instead of maladaptive ones (avoidance, excessive screen time).

Recovery Capacity

Regular physical activity enhances body's energy cells, improves energy efficiency in muscles, improving endurance and recovery rates for life's physical challenges.

Long-Term Social and Emotional Resilience

Long-term resilience in children and teenagers means having the mental and physical "reserve" to handle challenges, bounce back from setbacks, and adapt to change over months and years – not just in the short term.

Physical activity strengthens this reserve through sustained brain, body, and social adaptations and MUST be part of the paradigm for a happy and healthy life for children and teenagers alongside a nurturing and caring home environment and education.

Conclusion

In this book I have provided you with an extensive overview into the proven holistic and therapeutic benefits of physical activity in children and teenagers.

In addition, as the term physical activity suggests, it can be of any description of your choosing and will provide significant benefits – as it has done for me – provided it is undertaken three times or more per week.

This frequency of physical activity gives families plenty of time to incorporate many other activities of daily living comfortably whilst providing huge benefits in both the short and long term.

Physical activity does not have to be expensive; it just has to be regular; and as conclusively proven by the evidence, regular physical activity will go a long way to ensure that your children grow up with sound body, brain and character.

Now more than ever, given the screen demic, as well as the massive increase in the diagnosis of mental health conditions in children and teenagers, a ready made treatment in the form of regular Physical Activity is in your hands! Time to move!

CHAPTER 21

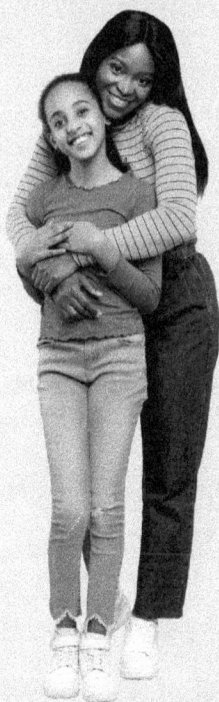

'FIVE A DAY'
YOUR TIPS FOR A HEALTHIER
SCREEN TIME

'How much is too much
screen time for children?'

'Studies have shown a clear
link between **excessive screen
time** and issues such as
delayed speech and **language
development, communication
difficulties, reduced
concentration spans, poor sleep**
and **mental health problems.**'

HEALTH PROFESSIONALS FOR SAFER SCREENS

SCAN ME

NHS Leicester Children's Hospital

Accepted by **NHS** England Mental Health Leads

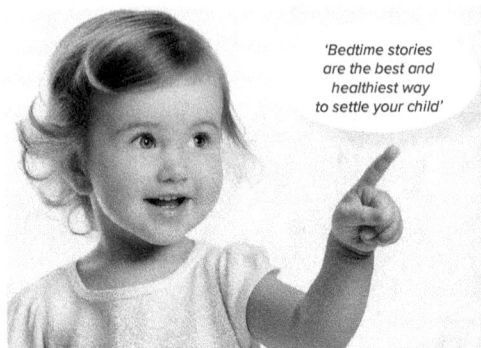

'Bedtime stories are the best and healthiest way to settle your child'

Birth to 5 years

'Studies have shown that too much screen time can cause babies and toddlers to learn fewer words and have slower language development. Excessive use of screens is also being strongly linked to behavioural difficulties in very young children.'

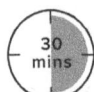

0-24 months

30 mins

2 - 5 year olds

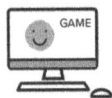

GAME

Bigger is better

Watching lots of short videos is being linked to concentration difficulties in children.

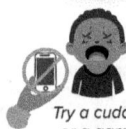

Try a cuddle or a game

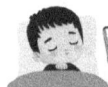

Phones, tablets and computers should not be in any child's bedroom overnight.

RECOMMENDATIONS:

1 **NO screen time** between **birth - 24 months** except for video chatting with family and friends.

2 **30 MINS screen time.** Children aged **2 - 5 years old** should not be on screens for more than **30 min per day.**

3 **BIGGER screens.** If your child is ready to **play a short game** then try to use a larger screen like a **tablet or computer screen.** These cause less visual strain than a phone.

4 **AVOID** using a device **to settle your child** down. Evidence shows this makes their anger and frustration worse in later life. **Instead try a book, a game outdoors, or just a cuddle.**

5 *SLEEP HYGIENE. Under 5's should **not use a screen** for at least **2 HOURS BEFORE BEDTIME,** to aid their natural sleep pattern.

* **'SLEEP HYGIENE'** is a term used for healthy habits and behaviours that help support a good night's sleep.

'Walk, run, ride a bike, anything that gets kids up and about and off their screens'

'Try and ensure screen-free time together'

Ditch screens at mealtimes! 'Studies show that eating in front of screens leads to higher obesity risk as children consume more unhealthy food!'

6 to 10 years

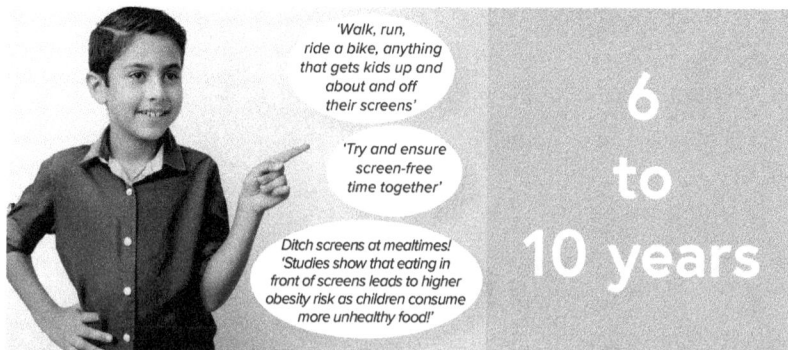

Studies show there is a clear link between excessive screen use and difficulties with concentration, sleep and mental health. There may also be distinct physical changes in the developing brain.'

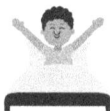

No screens

M	T	W	T	F	S	S

not more than 1-2hrs/day   up to 2hrs/day

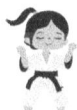

Keep active

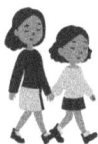

Screen-free time together

Reports suggest adults touch their phones over 2000 times a day.

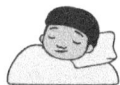

Sleep Hygiene. No screens 1 hour before bedtime

RECOMMENDATIONS:

1 **WAKING UP WITHOUT screens** It is recommended that social media/screens are not used for the first hour of the day.

2 **1-2 HRS PER DAY** is the suggested screen time in the week and not more than **2 hours on weekends.**

3 **STAY ACTIVE** Encourage physical activity for **1-2 hours a day.**

Watching lots of short videos on platforms such as TikTok and YouTube is being linked to concentration difficulties in children.

4 **SCREEN-FREE time together** Children will often mimic behaviours of the adults around them. **Consider your own social media usage/ phone checking behaviour.**

5 It is recommended that screens **should not be used 1 HOUR** before bedtime. **Phones, tablets and computers should not be in a bedroom overnight.**

* 'SLEEP HYGIENE' is a term used for healthy habits and behaviours that help support a good night's sleep.

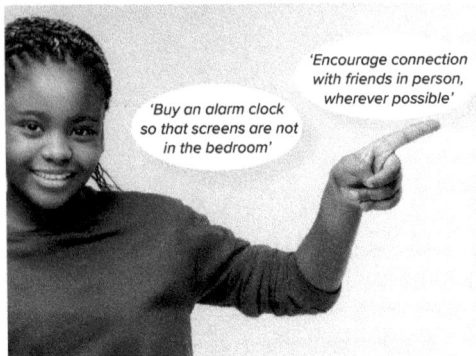

'Buy an alarm clock so that screens are not in the bedroom'

'Encourage connection with friends in person, wherever possible'

11 to 17 years

'Studies show there is a clear link between excessive social media and screen use and difficulties with concentration, sleep and mental health. There may also be distinct physical changes in the developing brain.'

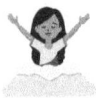

No screens

M	T	W	T	F	S	S
Up to 2hrs/day					Up to 2-3 hrs /day	

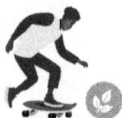

Stay active.
More green time,
less screen time

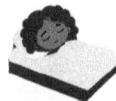

Screen-free
time together

No screens at least
1 hour before bedtime

RECOMMENDATIONS:

1 **WAKING UP WITHOUT screens** It is recommended that social media/screens are **not used for the first hour of the day.**

2 **SCREEN TIME** As a general rule, it is suggested that screen time **should not exceed 1-2 hours per day** in the week and not more than **3 hours on weekends.**

Watching lots of short videos on platforms such as TikTok and YouTube is being linked to concentration difficulties in children.

3 **STAY ACTIVE** Encourage physical activity for at least **an hour per day.**

4 **SCREEN-FREE time together** Children will often mimic behaviours of the adults around them. **Consider your own social media usage.**

Be careful of violent or frightening content especially before bed.

5 **Phones, tablets and computers should not be in a bedroom overnight.**

HEALTH PROFESSIONALS FOR SAFER SCREENS

.

www.ingramcontent.com/pod-product-compliance
Lightning Source LLC
Chambersburg PA
CBHW030020290326
41934CB00005B/415